Living Pain-free with **Osteoarthritis**

How I succeeded in putting my osteoarthritis into REMISSION and prevented surgery naturally

Printed in Great Britain by

remous print

Unit 4, Barton View Business Park, Sheeplands Lane
Sherborne, Dorset DT9 4FW

ACKNOWLEDGEMENTS

I would like to acknowledge the help of the following people in the making of this book:

> Dr Harriet F Collins, MBBS MRCGP MFSEM(UK), DRCOG DipSEM for her assessment of my condition and for permission to use her written report.
> Elaine Taylor, MA, MSocInd, for agreeing to be my model and for editing and proofreading the book.
> Alan Bunter of Remous Print Ltd for taking the manuscript, producing and printing my book to a professional standard.

Finally I would like to thank my lovely wife Justine not only for her help with the recipes but also for her patience, understanding and support while I have been engaged in writing.

TESTIMONIALS

At 12 years old I was told that I had hyper mobility of my joints. As a result of this I had already suffered multiple dislocations, mainly in my shoulders, knees and elbows. I was given braces, crutches, and had physiotherapy, including small electric shocks into my muscles and full leg casts, numerous times - all to no avail. I was offered surgery on my left knee at the age of 16 to take away scar tissue and tighten the muscles. I refused due to my age and being told that I would have a massive scar on my leg. This process was repeated until I reached the age of 20 when I was given more scans and again offered surgery. Unfortunately, at the pre-operation appointment I found out that I was pregnant and couldn't have the surgery. As the years went by, I found myself being so busy with children that I didn't have time to consider the surgery route anymore. Dislocations become worse, requiring ever more medical intervention. My hip was now dislocating too, along with other joints. I was again told surgery was my only option - to put a screw through my muscle into my bone and clear out the scar tissue. This is when I started looking for alternative answers.

Before having children I had trained with Kire for few months at his regular fitness classes and, in 2015, my children started martial arts training with him. I recalled him saying that he was self-helping with his osteo-arthritis so I asked if he would help me too and he agreed. The mission was on to strengthen my joints. Kire researched and showed me modified exercises and gave me diet advice. We trained 3-4 times a week and slowly but surely I became stronger. I noticed fewer problems with my joints. After a few months I went on a girls night out and, for the first time in years, I wore high heels without being in agony after a few hours. The training continued and my strength increased; I had no dislocations or pains at all. I have now been dislocation- and pain-free for several years. Without Kire I would have had multiple surgeries and so much more pain and suffering. I can't thank him enough for the hard work and dedication he put into my recovery and strengthening. He is, without a doubt, the most knowledgeable person about muscles and the body I have ever met.

Nicky Liddle

I experienced severe back pain for over two years, which prevented me from carrying out the sport of cycling which I had previously participated in. After several visits to the doctor, who prescribed tablets as a solution, and several, also weekly, visits to my chiropractor, there were no permanent results.

I met Kire at a local business networking group and told him about my back problems. He suggested a training programme and diet aimed at improving my core strength and flexibility to help repair my lower back injury. After only a few one-to-one training sessions I started to feel the benefits. I continued to train with Kire and, with his guidance, I returned to normal within six months with no pain in my back. This allowed me to return to my sport of cycling. The knowledge Kire has is outstanding and I still continue to carry out several of the exercises he taught me and follow the recommended diet to prevent any possible future injuries.

Matthew Williams

My life was hectic and, with both a family and a business, stressful. I was suffering with depression and life was a struggle. I had also been under investigation for some chest pains. My wife Hayley, who suffered for a few months with a lower back problem, met Kire at our local garage. He suggested to her that he may be able to help her and she signed up for a one-hour, one-to-one private fitness lesson once a week. A few weeks later we agreed that I too should give it a go and so I signed up for one-to-one lessons twice a week. Kire took all that I had to say about depression and life into account and worked on my fitness, including a weak shoulder and back which had arisen after a nasty accident some years before. Ongoing investigations into my chest pains showed that I had vascular disease, with a high chance of needing several stents.

Kire created programmes for me with diet suggestions and, after three months of training for one hour twice a week, cutting down on alcohol and adjusting my diet, I felt so different. Then the day arrived for my angiogram. The results showed that I didn't need the stents; what a relief! I was told to carry on doing whatever it was that I was doing, as it was obviously making a difference. Our health in general improved greatly, my wife no longer having problems with her lower back. Despite still having vascular disease, I don't need stents, my shoulder and back are much better and neither of them give me any problems. My depression is in check and the world is a lot brighter. My family can't thank Kire enough.

Stuart Hurford

For many years I played rugby at a high level with the commensurate damage to my joints and muscles that restricted true mobility and flexibility. I have had over a dozen operations on my joints as a result of osteoarthritis caused by damage and wear and tear. This has previously degraded my quality of life and the enjoyment of many activities due to the pain and discomfort I experienced with mobility. I first met Kire when I thought perhaps martial arts would be an engaging activity that I could do within the limits of my joint problems. The flexibility, mobility and comfort I have been able to achieve since following his inspirational programme has been nothing short of life-changing. I have been able to fully engage with all aspects of martial arts, have achieved ranges of movement and agility not previously experienced and what was a progressive degeneration of mobility has been halted in its tracks. From the warm-up to the warm-down each exercise specifically targets joint structure to increase mobility, strengthen structure and subsequently ease discomfort. Coupled with a carefully considered nutrition plan this system is perfect for anyone suffering joint problems with osteoarthritis. I cannot recommend it enough. You really can live pain-free.

Gary Stubbs

Contents

INTRODUCTION

Most commonly called degenerative joint disease, osteoarthritis (OA) is the most common chronic condition of the joints. In the UK, more than 9 million people have osteoarthritis. In England and Wales, there are approximately 160,000 hip and knee replacement procedures performed each year. (*www.njrcentre.org.uk*)

OA is a condition that causes joints to become painful and stiff. OA can affect any joint of the fingers, toes, knees, hips, lower back, neck and shoulders.

As part of normal life, our joints are exposed to a constant low level of damage. In most cases the body repairs the damage itself and, in the beginning, we don't experience any symptoms. However, with continual use of our joints, the cartilage lining starts to roughen and thin out, and our tendons and ligaments must work harder. While normal joints will have cartilage that provides a smooth, gliding surface for joint motion and acts as a cushion between the bones, with OA the joints lose the cartilage which breaks down, causing pain, swelling and problems moving the joint. This can lead to the formation of bony spurs called osteophytes. The area can become inflamed, red and swollen. Severe loss of cartilage can lead to bone rubbing on bone, altering the shape of the joint and forcing the bones out of their normal position.

The exact cause of OA isn't known but several things are thought to increase your risk of developing OA: overusing a joint following joint injury and before the joint is fully healed; age; family history; and obesity.

ABOUT THIS BOOK

I have written this book with the intention of helping fellow martial arts practitioners and fitness industry professionals like myself, as well as runners, walkers, body builders, dancers and gymnasts. Also, people who perform heavy lifting in their work environment and others that suffer from wear and tear of their hip joints, and of course other joints too.

In our everyday life, from a very early age, we use our joints constantly – some more than others, depending on our lifestyle. Our joints are exposed to low levels of damage, although, in most cases, our body should repair the damage itself without our experiencing any symptoms.

The exact reason why osteoarthritis develops is unknown, however several things are thought to increase the risk of it developing:

- **Joint injury**: overusing our joints after injury or operation without giving them time to self-repair
- **Overweight** (obesity): being very overweight puts excessive strain on our joints, particularly those that bear most of our weight (hips and knees)
- **Age**: our risk of developing osteoarthritis increases as we get older
- **Family history**: osteoarthritis may run in families, although studies are not conclusive.

Knowing this, is there something we can do to prevent OA developing or, in the early stage of the disease, try to stop or slow down the development of this life-changing condition?

I was diagnosed with severe osteoarthritis in 2011 and suffered for a few years with both pain and uncertainty – would I need a hip replacement operation? Would I need to change my lifestyle and give up my martial arts career? I spent much time exploring this disease and experimenting with different exercises and diet plans. Finally, I have the confidence and knowledge to write this book, in the hope of either helping people to prevent OA from developing or, for those who have already developed OA, to help them put it in remission and live a relatively pain-free, fit life. Like myself, there are many athletes who enjoy a life of fitness, having trained from a young age in the belief that keeping fit was enough to prevent most health problems, especially joint problems, from occurring. However, they are not necessarily preventing the joints from developing this painful condition.

All exercises given in this book have been carefully created and selected after years of development and experimentation. They have helped not only me but also some of my students with joint problems, including OA. From my experience, exercises alone are not enough without a good diet plan. I have created my own over many years following my OA diagnosis and I end this book with some advice on food to include in your diet and some interesting recipes.

TREATING OSTEOARTHRITIS - OA

OA can't be cured but I believe its development can be slowed down or stopped, putting it in remission. It is possible to regain flexibility and movement in your joints and hopefully, like me, you will be left pain-free.

This can be achieved by losing weight, changing your diet by increasing the amount of anti-inflammatory foods you eat, avoiding inflammatory food and regular, correctly performed strengthening and stretching exercises to maintain mobility in the muscles around the joints and their ligaments and tendons.

My personal belief from my own experience with OA is that it might be possible to prevent OA with correct diet and correct exercises. It is now 9 years since I was diagnosed with OA in my hips and, by following a specific exercise programme and anti-inflammatory diet, I have managed to stop the progress of OA – to put it in remission – and regain some of my previous mobility. I am now pain-free in my hips.

If I had known years ago what I know now and had done the exercise programme and diet I have developed and practiced since my diagnosis, it may be that I would never have developed OA in my hips or any other joints in the first place.

PROFESSIONAL REPORT

Professional report about the progress I have made with my hips, following a consultation, examination, and study of my X-rays

Kire reports in this book about his personal journey dealing with painful osteoarthritis of his hips. He had painful very limited osteoarthritis of the hips confirmed on his first x-ray in 2011.

At this time he was recommended by his regular Dr at his GPs, to take high-dose analgesia with referral for early hip replacements. However, with the active life he has led and his desire to continue with the martial arts coaching, he was aware that he may not be able to continue with this after his hip replacements. He therefore developed his own stretching, exercise programme and dietary plan to try to help which has, over the last 7 years, resulted in PAIN FREE functional hips, allowing him to still teach and demonstrate martial arts and fitness at his academy.

Having examined Kire recently, there is no doubt that he still has limitation due to reduced joint space in both hips. He still has an adjusted gait due to restriction but he is pain-free in functional activities. His x-ray has also not changed in the intervening years (*see images*).

Kire has worked on flexibility with specific passive stretching machines as well as passive and isometrics floor stretching to help with this. He has excellent strength around the hips girdle that has been maintained with his exercises plan. He has careful weight control though diet but he has also adjusted his diet significantly to follow an 'anti-inflammatory' protocol.

Kire has managed to keep the range of movement and symptoms in his hips well controlled with his stretching routine, exercises and anti-inflammatory diet. His x-rays remain unchanged a further 18 months on, a testament to excellent self-management.

Kire will present his journey as a personal case history in this book.

As a sport and exercise physician, I'm interested in way that people can maintain fitness and mobility with using exercise and a holistic approach including dietary considerations for good health, recovering and healing. Kire has shown personal resolve and determination to make a difference to his condition of severe osteoarthritis of his hips by his multi-faceted approach and others may benefit from a similar programme.

The next step would be to test this regime in others ideally under research guidelines.

Dr Harriet F Collins,
MBBS MRCGP MFSEM(UK), DRCOG DipSEM
GMC2932019
Sport & Exercise Medicine Doctor

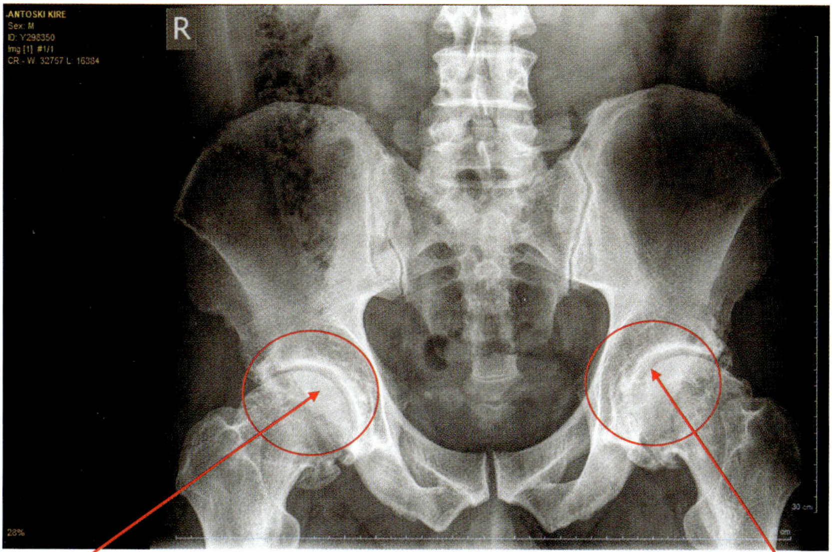

X - Ray March 2011

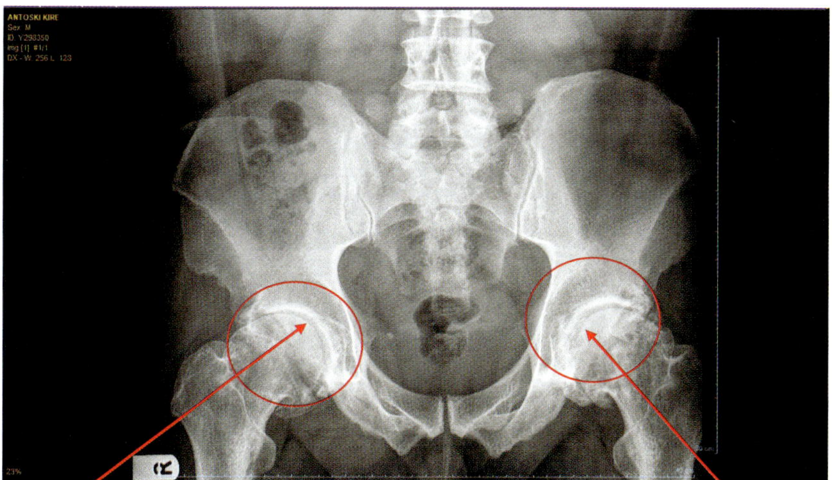

X - Ray December 2017

EXERCISE PROGRAMME

This exercise programme is suitable for practice at home or at the gym

The full exercise programme should be done regularly 2 to 3 times per week with a minimum of 48 hours rest between sessions

This workout, including 10 to 15 minutes' warm-up, can be done to your own dance music. Please choose something which has a beat ranging from 120bpm to 170bpm depending on your physical abilities and the speed at which you can do the exercises to the beat of the music.
If any of the exercises give you discomfort or pain, you can modify that exercise.

Prior to any physical activity, **warm-up** and **stretching** are very important.

- **Warm-up** is designed to raise body temperature and loosen up the muscles, in order to avoid injuries (pulled muscles or ruptured ligaments or tendons)
- **Stretching** is designed to loosen the body for better mobility.

AS WITH ANY EXERCISE PROGRAMME, IF YOU ARE UNSURE OF YOUR ABILITY TO PERFORM THE EXERCISES PLEASE CONSULT A DOCTOR BEFORE BEGINNING

Pre-workout warm-up exercises

Pre-workout warm-up exercises are designed to gently raise body temperature and loosen up the muscles and joints to avoid injuries (pulled muscles or ruptured ligaments or tendons). They prepare the body for the more dynamic warm-up before stretching.

To warm up and loosen up the shoulders

- Put both hands on your hips ***(Figure 1)*** and rotate your shoulders forward, hunching your back as you do so ***(Figure 2).*** Hold for 5 seconds. Rotate your shoulders backwards, opening out your chest ***(Figure 3).*** Hold for 5 seconds. Repeat 4 times each way.

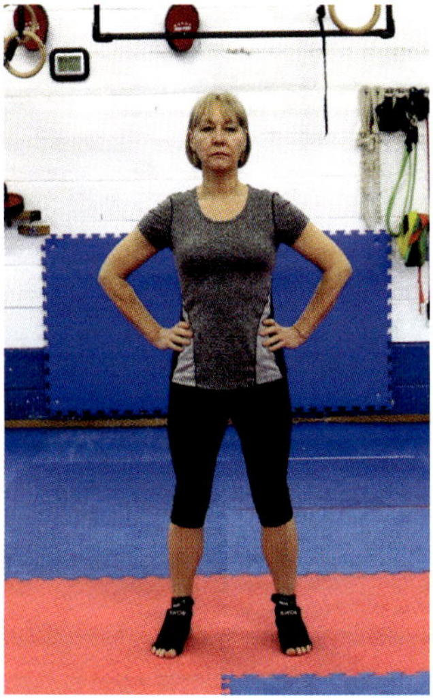

Figure 1

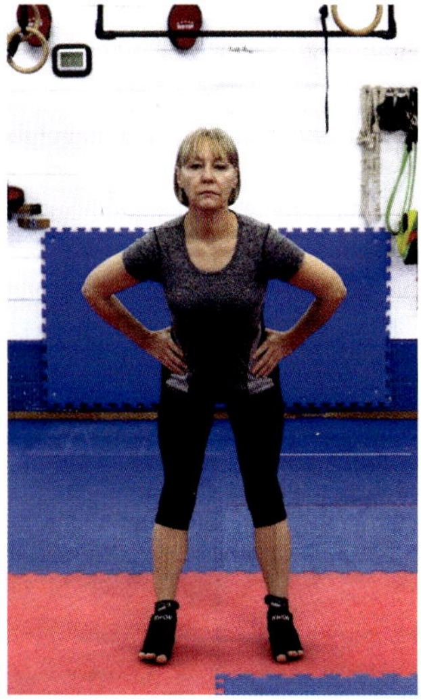

Figure 2

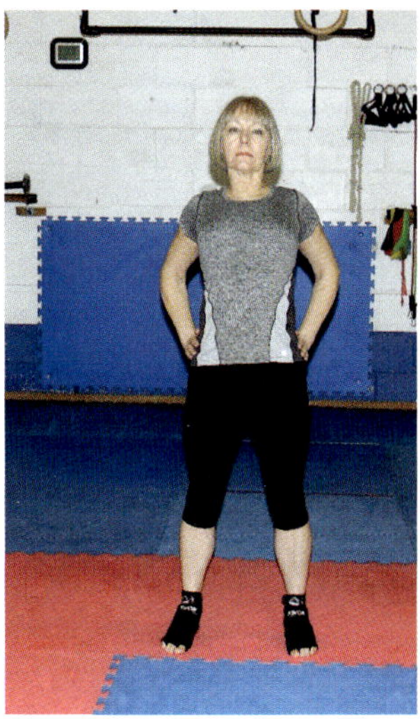

Figure 3

To warm up and loosen the elbows and wrist

- Lift your arms up to the side at shoulder-level and bend your arms at the elbows, rotate both forearms and wrist in a slow circular motion to the inside and outside. Repeat 4 times ***(Figures 4, 5 & 6).***

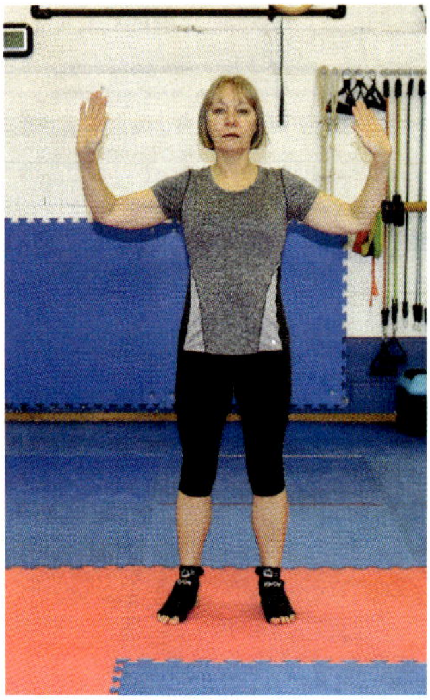

Figure 4

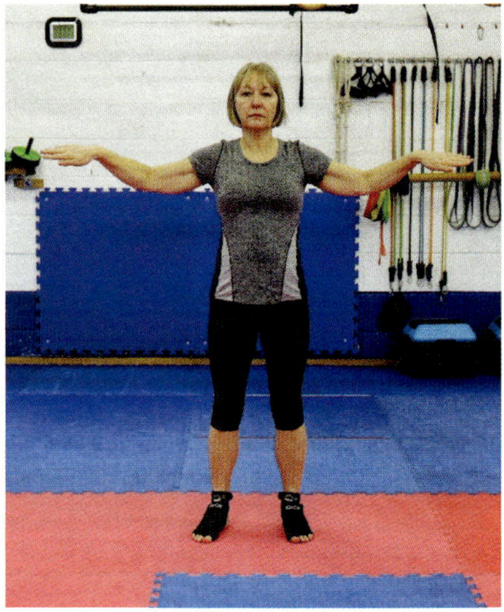

Figure 5

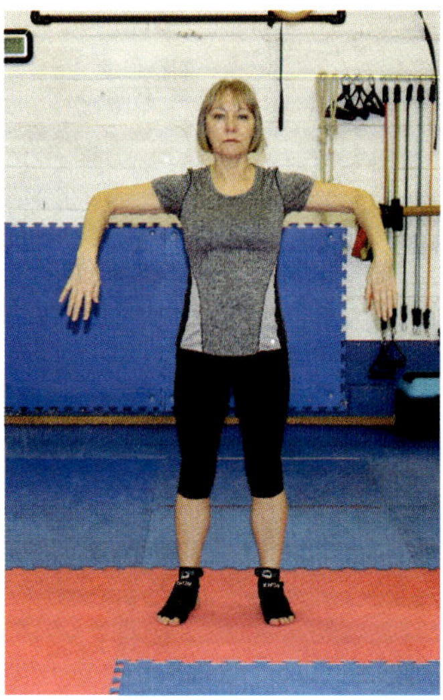

Figure 6

To warm up and loosen the back muscles

- Lift your arms out in front of you, shoulder height, with palms facing upwards. Swing your hands up and to the left, twisting at the waist and raising the right heel off the ground when turning. Follow your arms with your eyes, raising both hands over the left shoulder ***(Figure 7 side view).***
- Repeat to the right shoulder ***(Figure 8 side view).***
- Lower your hands down to the hips and repeat the move, turning first to the left hip ***(Figure 9)*** and then the right hip ***(Figure 10).***
- Repeat this exercise 4 times.

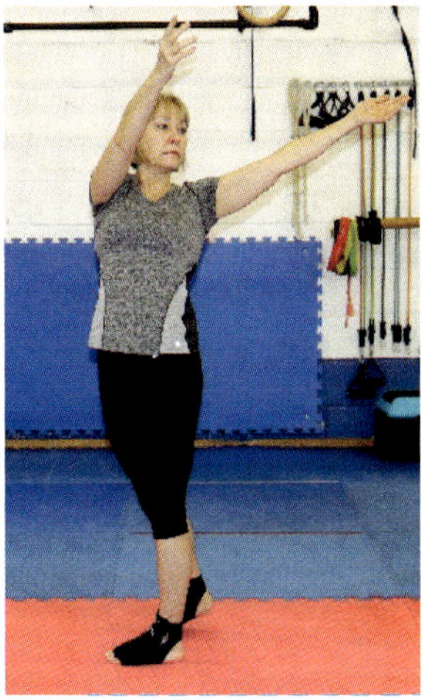

Figure 7 (side view)

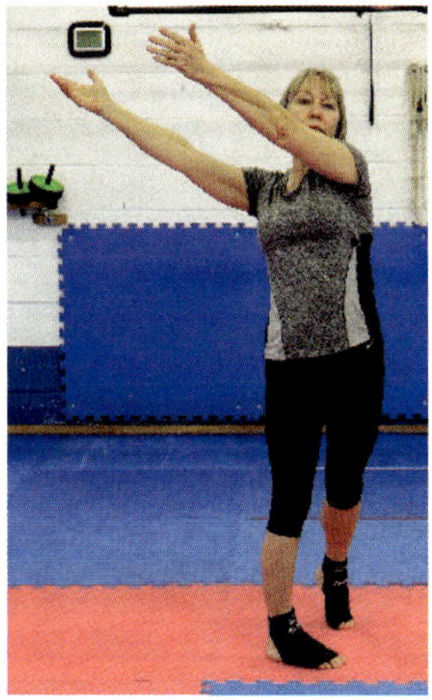

Figure 8 (side view)

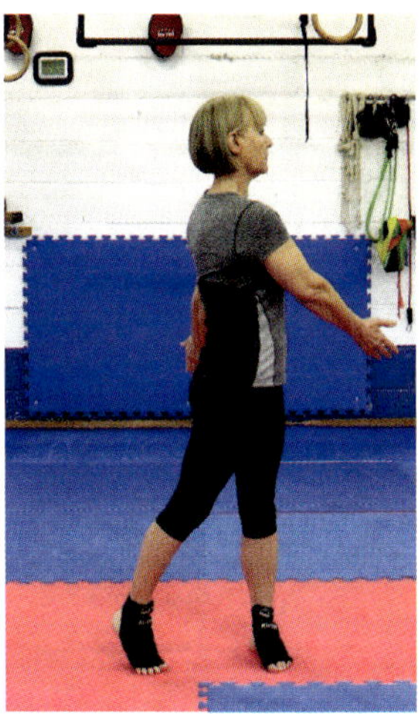

Figure 9

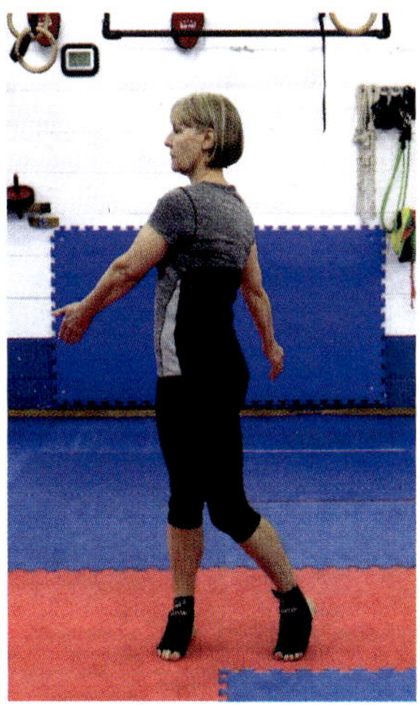

Figure 10

To warm up and loosen the hips

- Place your hands on your hips and rotate them in slow motion round to the left x 4 and then to the right x 4 ***(Figures 11, 12 & 13).***

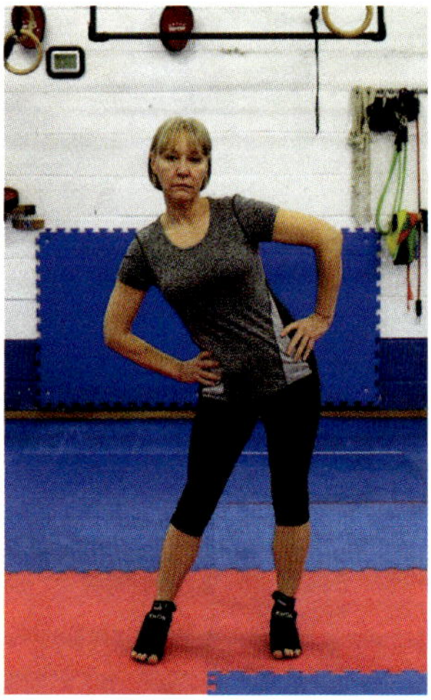

Figure 11

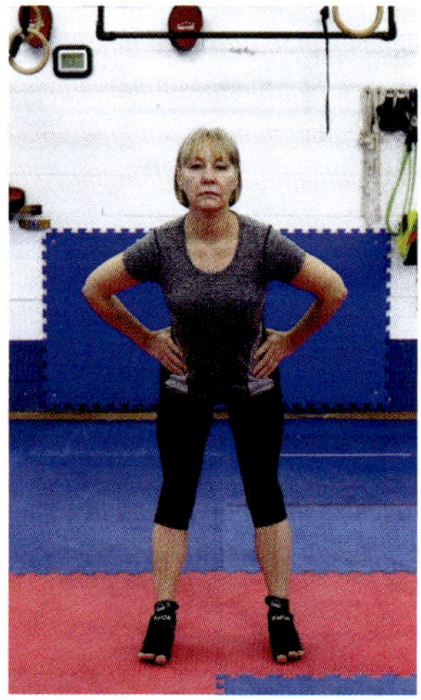

Figure 12

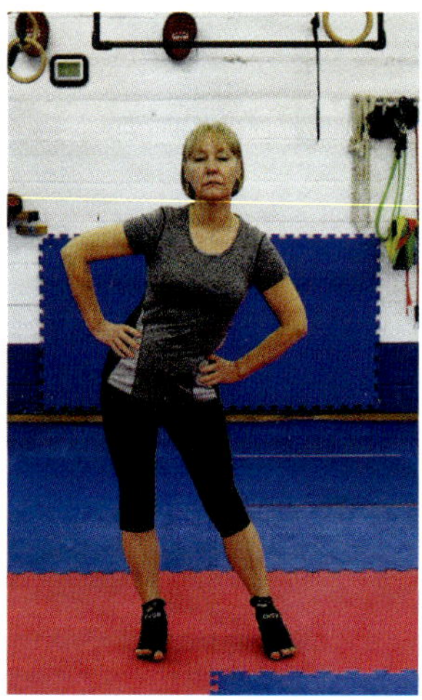

Figure 13

To warm up and loosen the knees

- Open your feet 30cm apart and place your hands on your knees. Rotate your knees inwards and outwards in slow motion x 4 ***(Figures 14 & 15).***

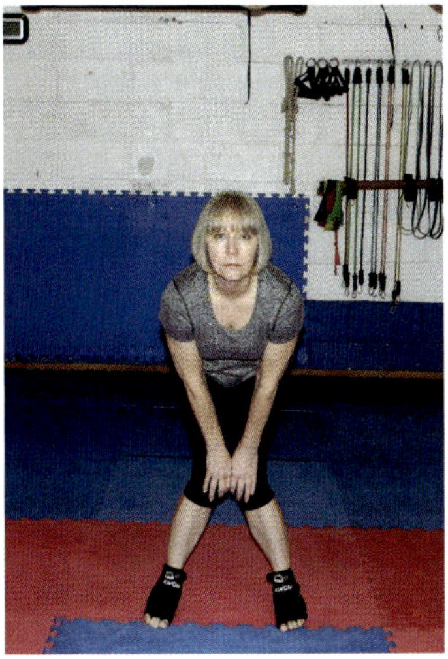

Figure 14

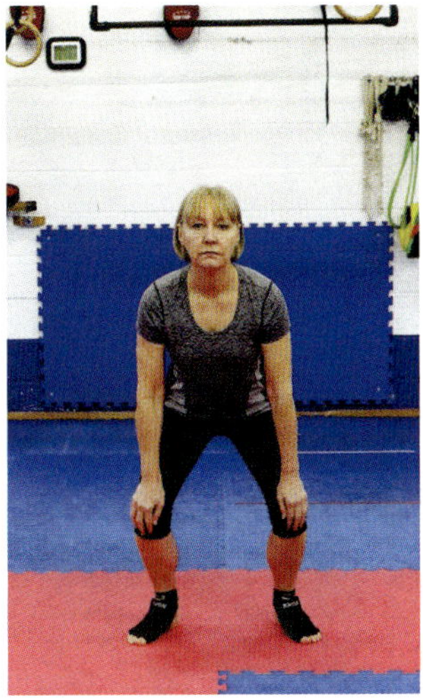

Figure 15

To warm up and loosen the neck muscles

- Take your right hand round the back and hold it with your left hand on your left hip. Gently bend your neck towards the left shoulder. Hold for 5-10 seconds ***(Figure 16).*** Repeat to the right side ***(Figure 17).***
- Stretch your hands out in front of you, thumbs up ***(Figure 18)*** and turn your head to the left side as if trying to look behind you. Hold for 5 -10 seconds ***(Figure 19).*** Repeat to the right side ***(Figure 20).***

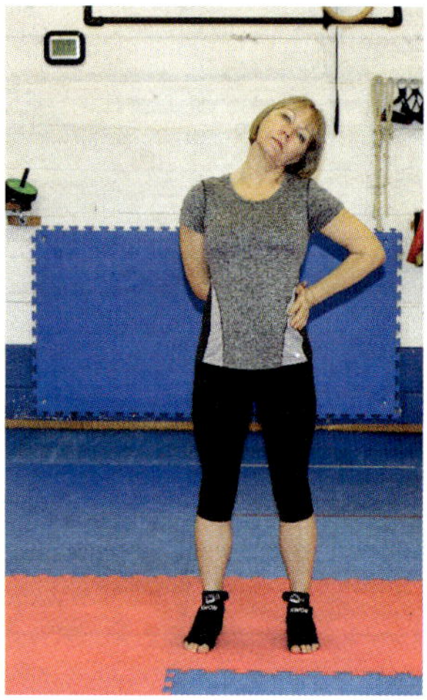

Figure 16

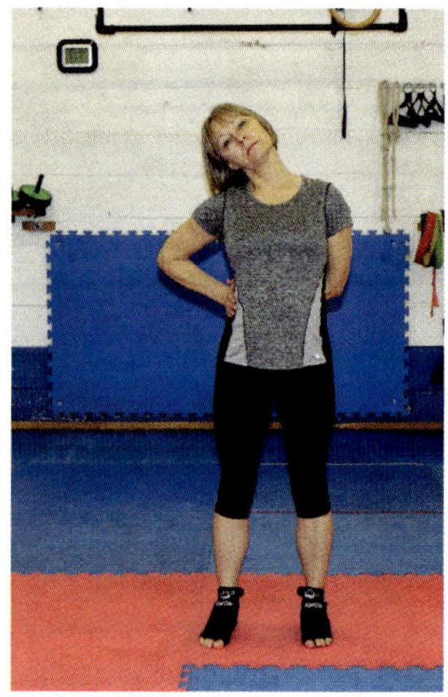

Figure 17

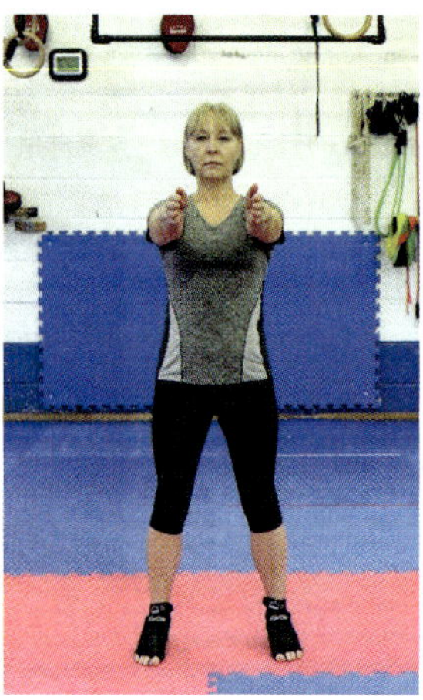

Figure 18

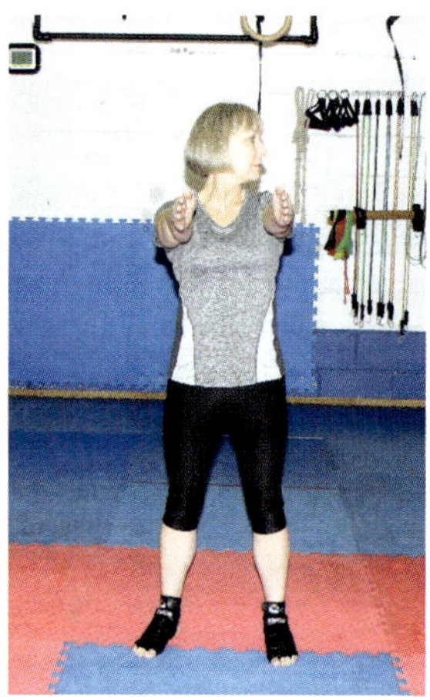

Figure 19

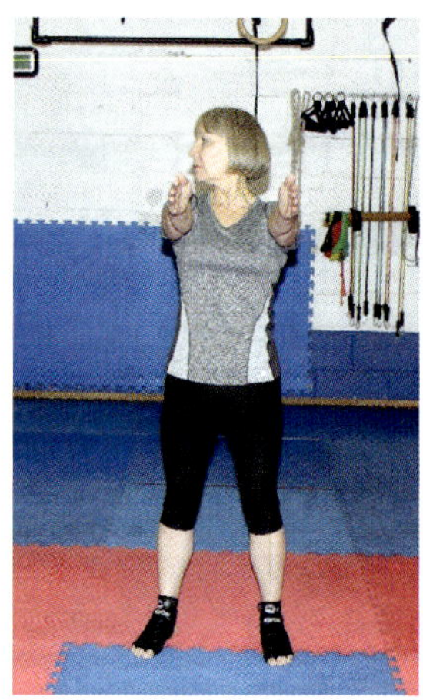

Figure 20

To warm up and loosen up hamstrings

- Gentle, forward, straight leg raises. Lift your left leg straight out in front of you, kicking up towards your left shoulder. Repeat 10 times ***(Figure 21 side view)***.
- Repeat with the right leg, 10 times ***(Figure 22 side view)***.

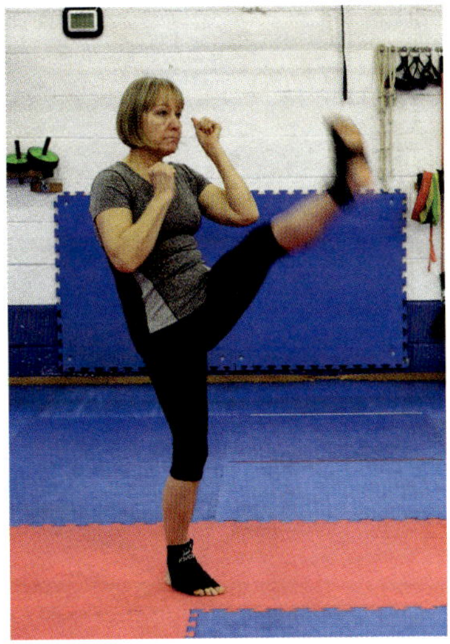

Figure 21 (side view)

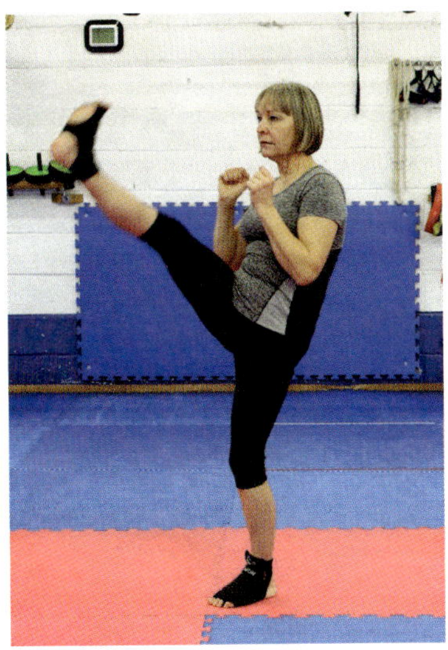

Figure 22 (side view)

Dynamic warm-up exercises

Dynamic warm-up exercises are designed to raise body temperature and heat up and loosen muscles and joints prior to stretching and high intensity work in order to avoid injuries (pulled muscles or ruptured ligaments or tendons).

Do the following exercises for 30 seconds each

To warm-up and loosen the hips and hip flexors

Knee raises

- Raise your left knee to your left shoulder x 4 ***(Figure 23).*** Then, in a jumping or static motion, cross your legs in front of you x 4, alternating left and right to the front ***(Figures 24 & 25).***
- Repeat with the right knee ***(Figure 26).***
- Repeat the exercise for 30 seconds.

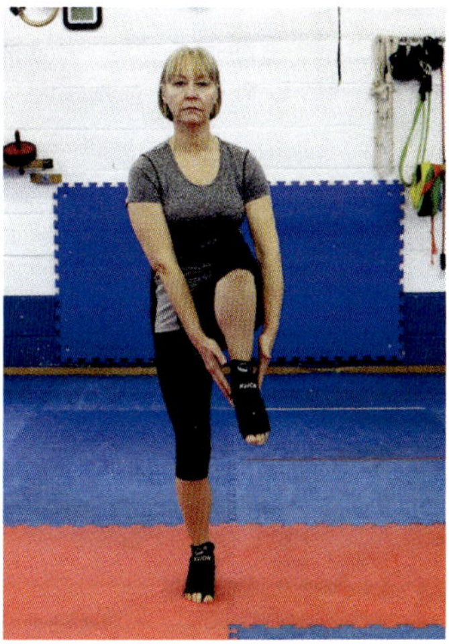

Figure 23

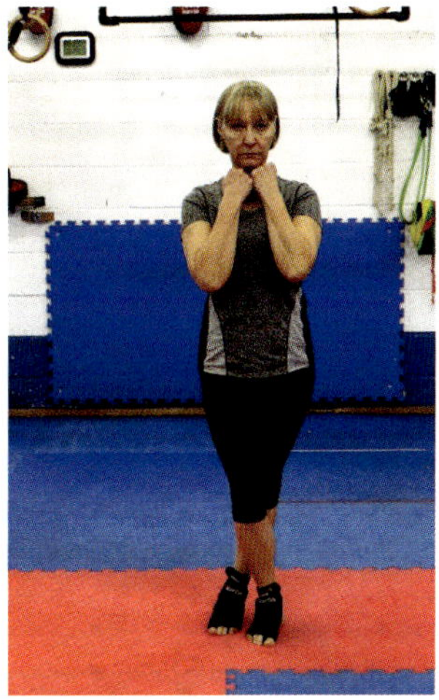

Figure 24

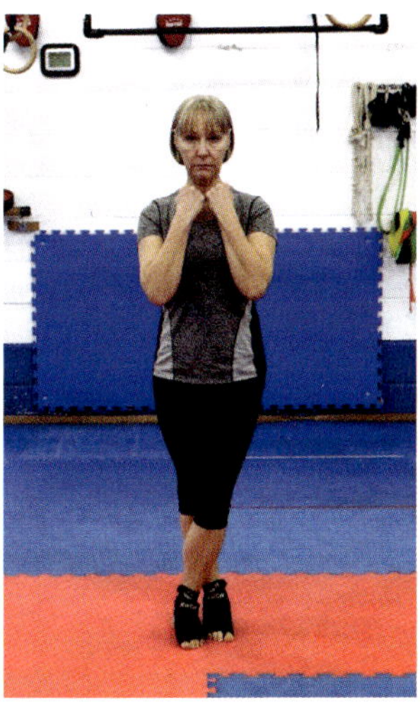

Figure 25

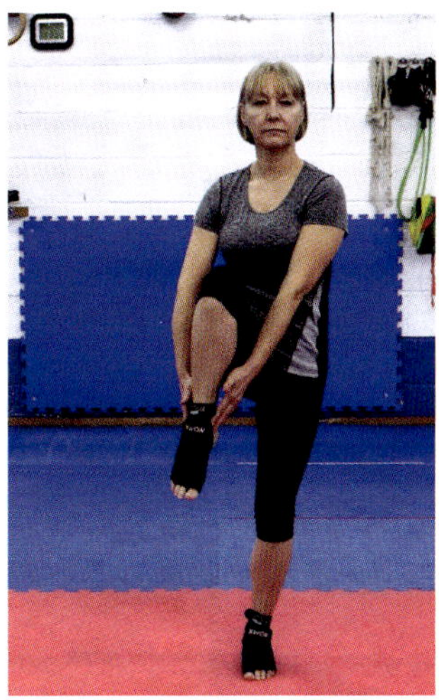

Figure 26

Back kicks

- Put your hands on your glutes ***(bottom)*** and kick your heels back up to your hands, alternating left leg and right leg ***(Figures 27 & 28 side view).***

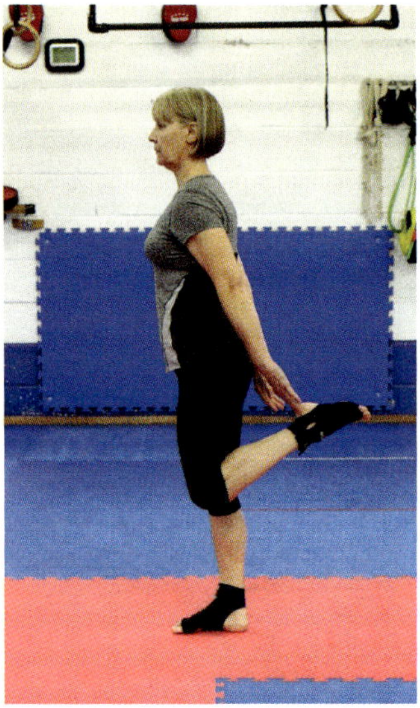

Figure 27 (side view)

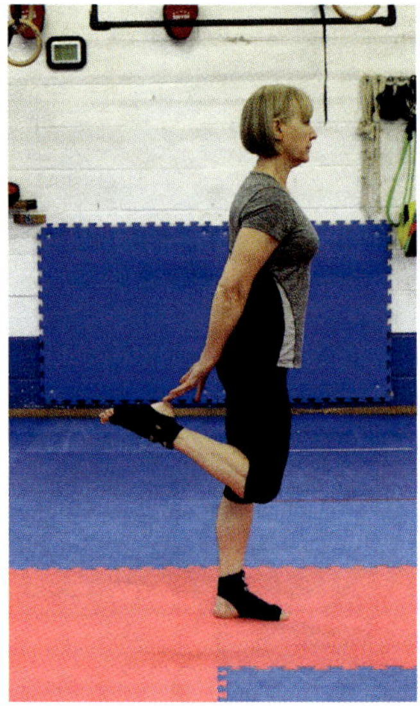

Figure 28 (side view)

Switch leg stance punching

- Raise your hands in the boxing guard ***(lift your hands up in front of your chin, elbows close to your body, and make a fist with both hands. Bend the fingers first and put the thumb over the fingers – do not put your thumb inside the fingers).***
- Put your left leg on the front and right leg back and extend your right hand ***(Figure 29).*** Then simultaneously switch them so that your right leg is on the front and the left hand is punching ***(Figure 30).***

Do not fully extend your arms at the elbow when punching

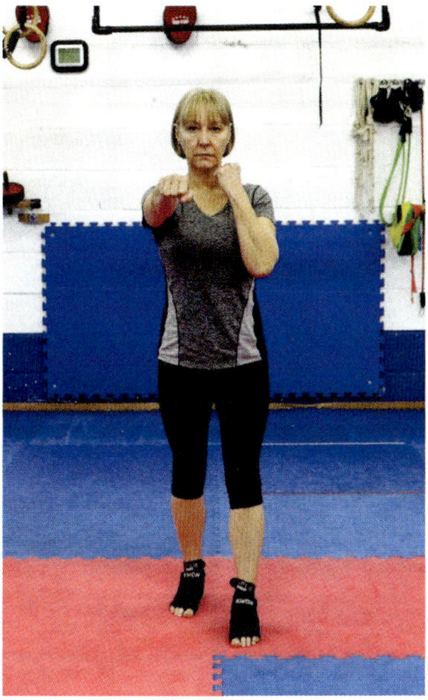

Figure 29

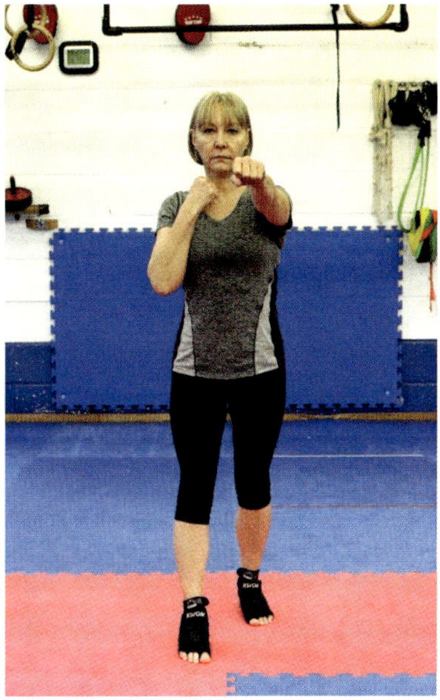

Figure 30

Squat and uppercut

- In a standing position, put your right hand in ***(boxing)*** uppercut position ***(Figure 31).*** Now jump to a wide, low squat, putting your palms on your knees *(**Figure 32**)*. Jump up with legs straight and feet together, this time putting your left hand in uppercut position ***(Figure 33).*** Again jump to a wide, low squat, putting your palms on your knees ***(Figure 34).*** Repeat for 30 seconds.

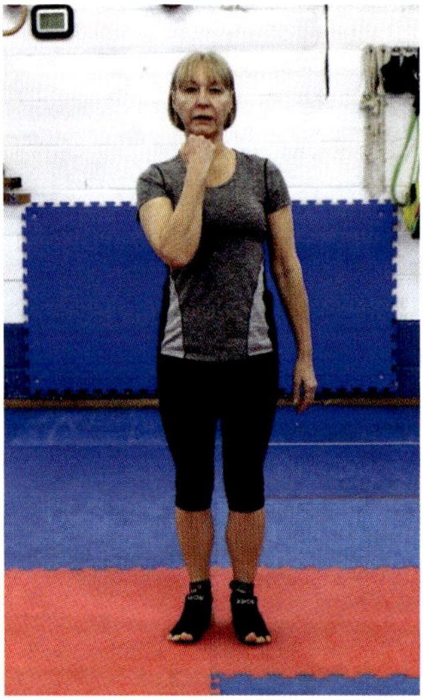

Figure 31

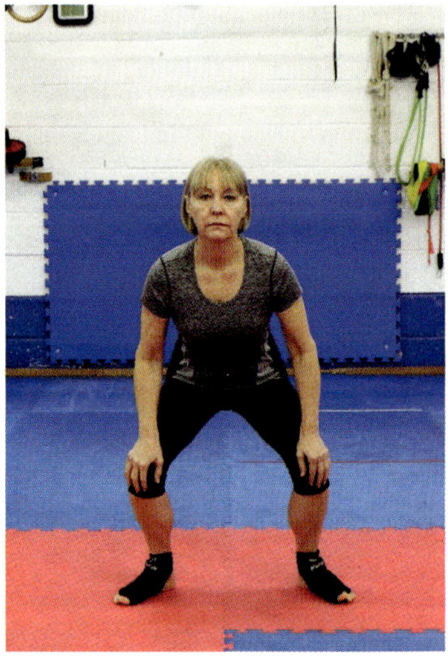

Figure 32

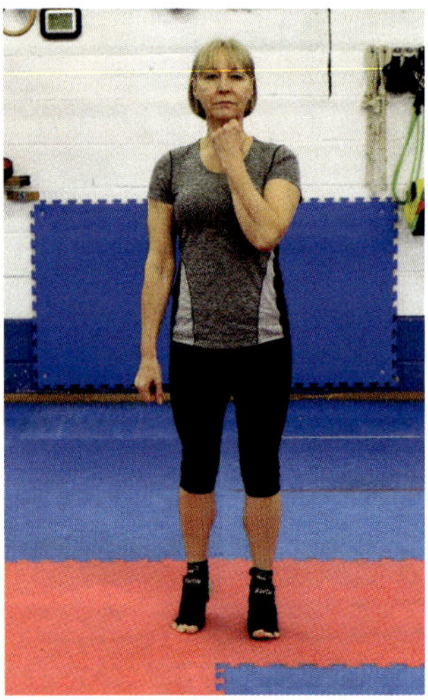

Figure 33

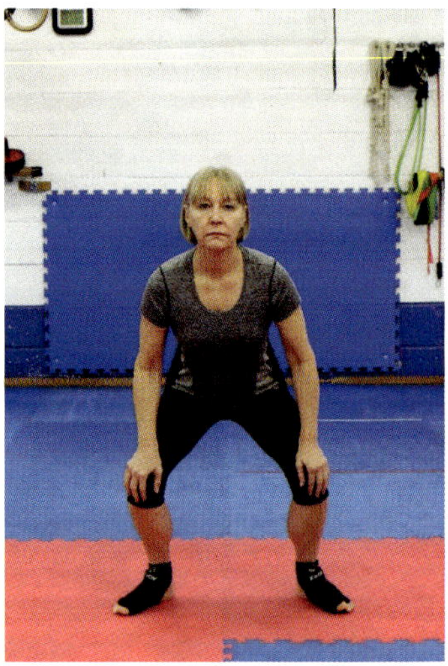

Figure 34

Side jumps

- Clasp your hands together and hold them on the front of your left hip ***(Figure 35).*** With feet together, hop to the left side, at the same time moving your hands to the right hip ***(Figure 36).***
- Repeat to the right side by moving your hands to the left hip.
- Continue with this exercise for 30 seconds.

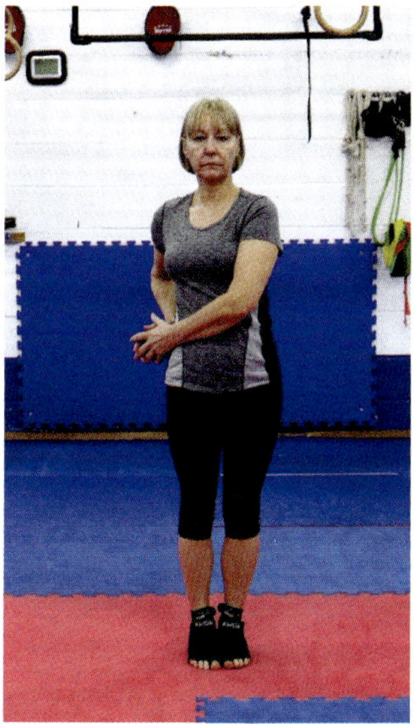

Figure 35

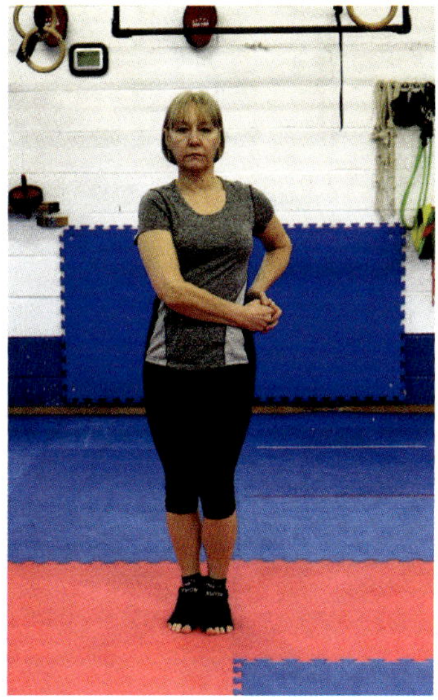

Figure 36

Lowering wide squats with punching

- From a standing position, extend your right arm in front of you, keeping your left hand to your chest ***(Figure 37).*** Gradually move forward, switching your hands in a striking motion in four stages, lowering the squats and opening your legs wider ***(Figures 38 & 39).*** Finally, gently punch the floor first with your left and then with your right hand ***(Figures 40 & 41).***
- Gradually move backwards in four stages ***(reversing Figures 38 & 39)*** returning to standing position ***(Figure 37).*** Repeat 4 times, depending on your fitness level.

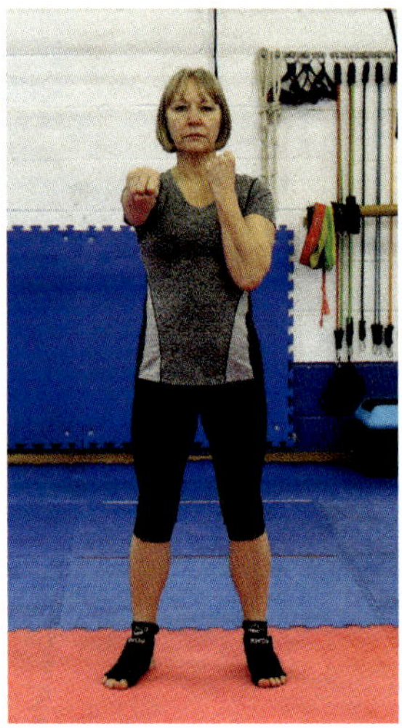

Figure 37

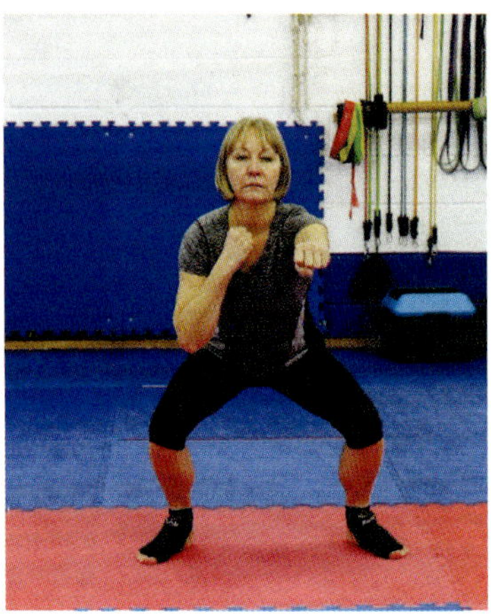

Figure 38

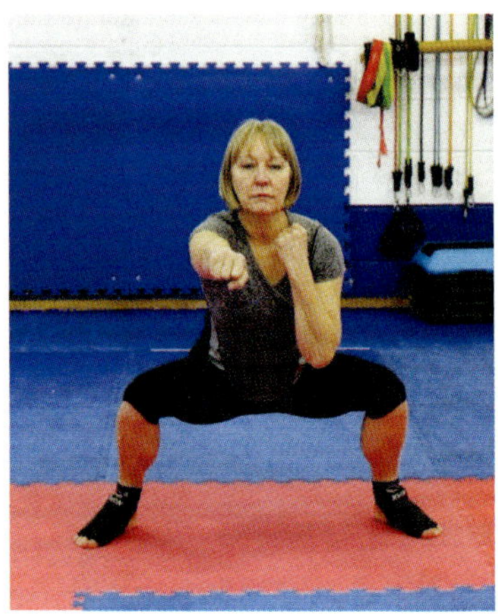

Figure 39

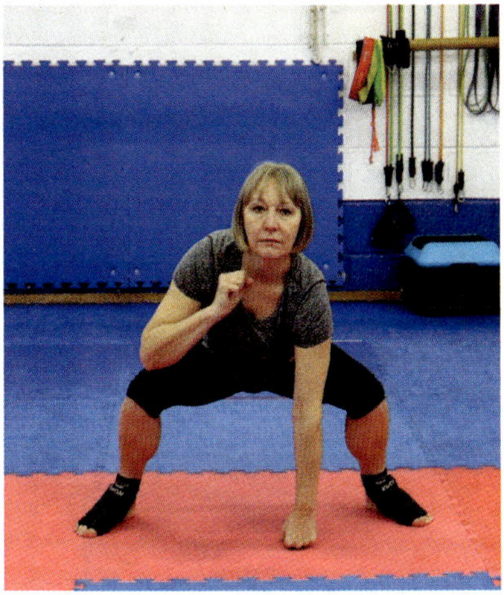

Figure 40

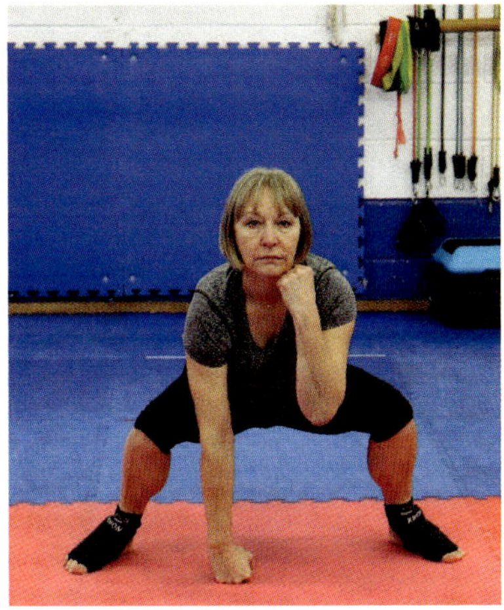

Figure 41

Rest for 30 seconds following the above exercises and before moving on.

Stretching

Stretching MUST be done prior to any dynamic work out to avoid temporary or permanent muscle and joint injuries

Static stretching must always be done in fully relaxed mode.

To loosen up and stretch hamstrings and adductors

- Breathing deeply through your nose, raise your hands above your head and hold your breath for 10-20 seconds ***(Figure 42).***
- Open your legs 30cm apart. As you slowly breathe out, squat deep with your heels on the floor and hold for 10-15 seconds ***(Figure 43).***
- Stand up and repeat, taking a deep breath through your nose and raising your hands above your head. Hold your breath for 10-20 seconds ***(Figure 44).***
- Open your legs a bit wider. Put your palms together and, breathing out, squat deep with your heels on the floor. Push your knees away with your elbows ***(Figure 45).***
- Stand up and open your legs to a comfortable box splits, with feet parallel and flat on the floor. Lower your body down between your legs and rest your palms on the floor ***(Figure 46)*** or, if you can, rest your elbows on the floor in front of you for a better stretch ***(Figure 47)***. Hold for 10-15 seconds.
- Move both hands to the left foot, or as near as you can, trying to reach your left foot with your right hand. Hold for 10-15 seconds ***(Figure 48).*** Then move your hands to the right leg and repeat the stretch ***(Figure 49).***
- Return to the centre position, rest your palms or elbows on the floor again ***(Figures 50 & 51)*** and widen your legs to your maximum comfortable stretch.

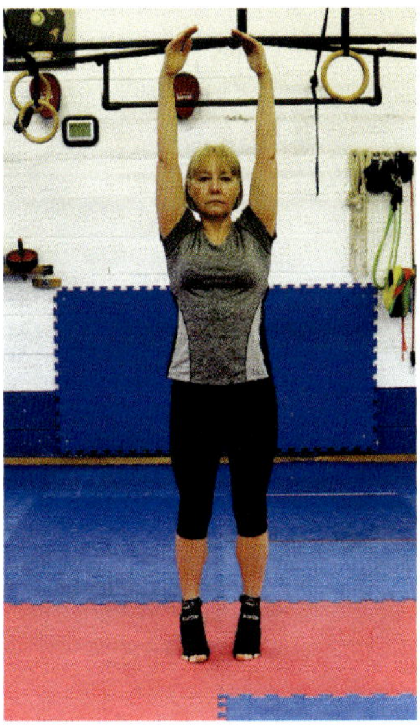

Figure 42

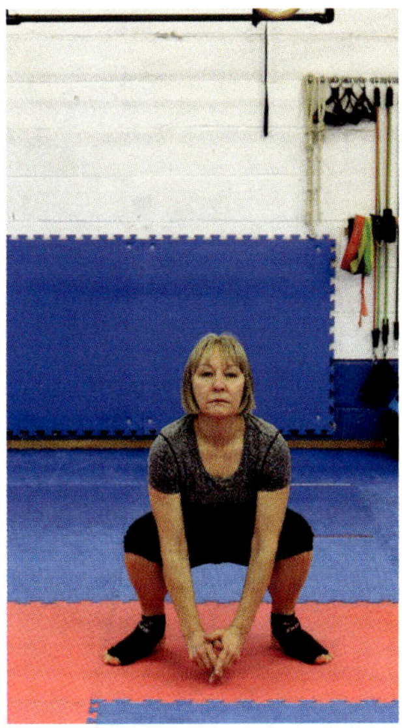

Figure 43

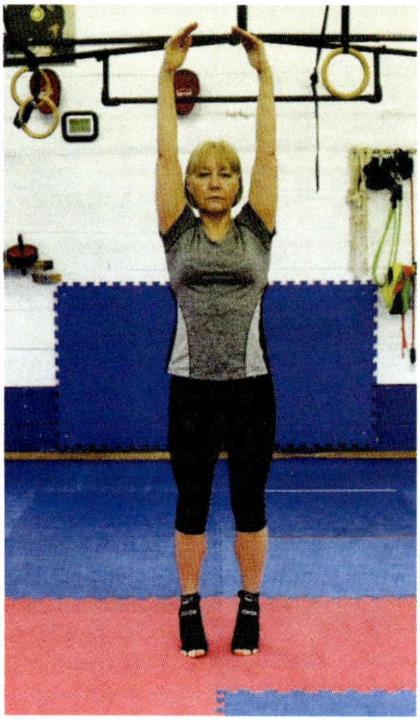

Figure 44

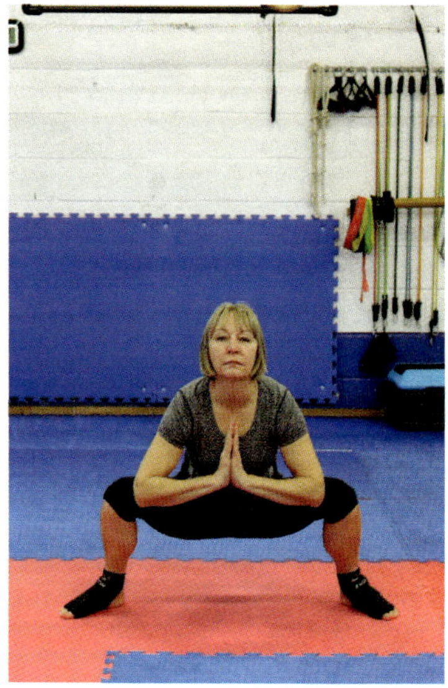

Figure 45

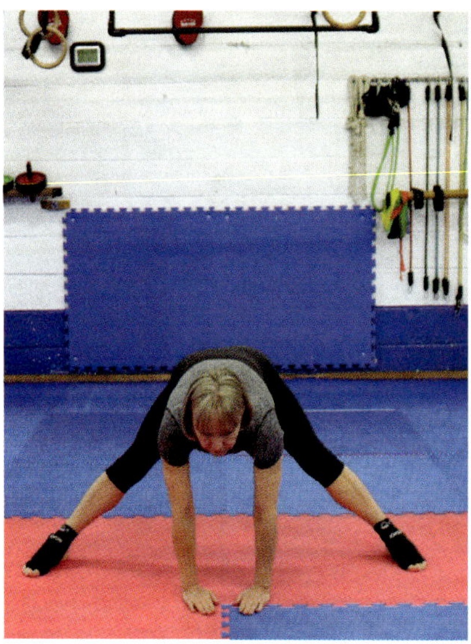

Figure 46

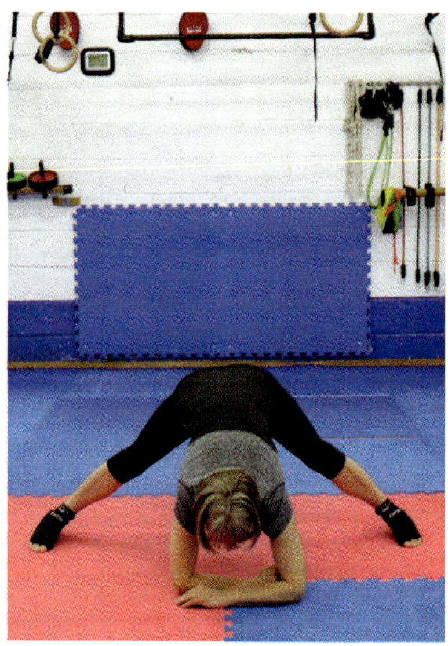

Figure 47

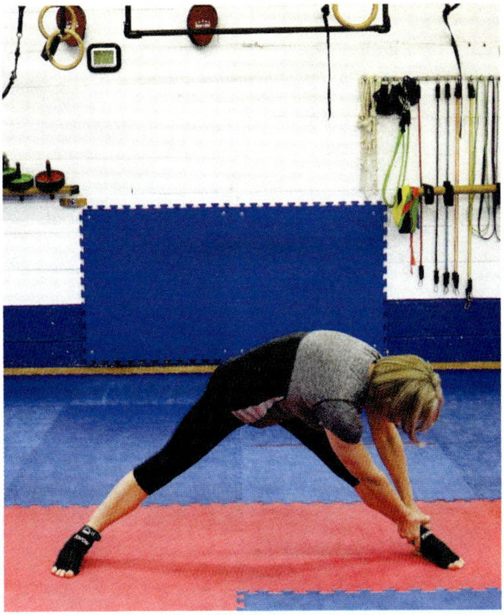

Figure 48

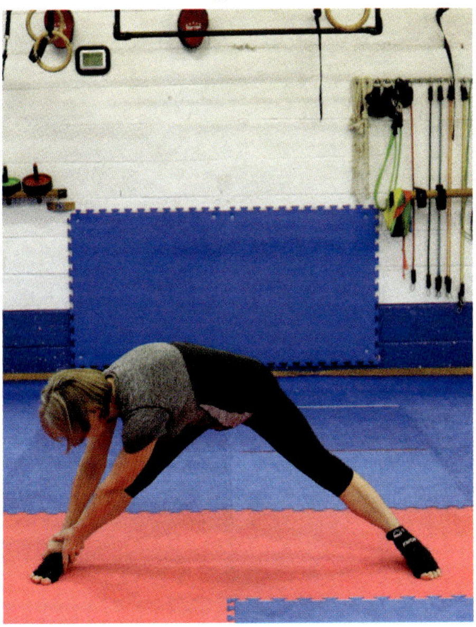

Figure 49

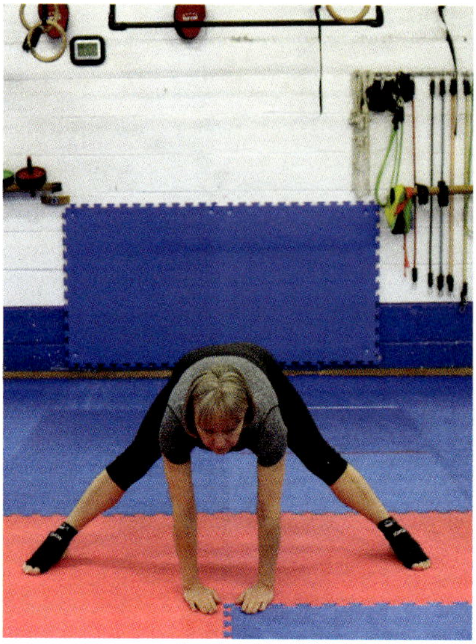

Figure 50

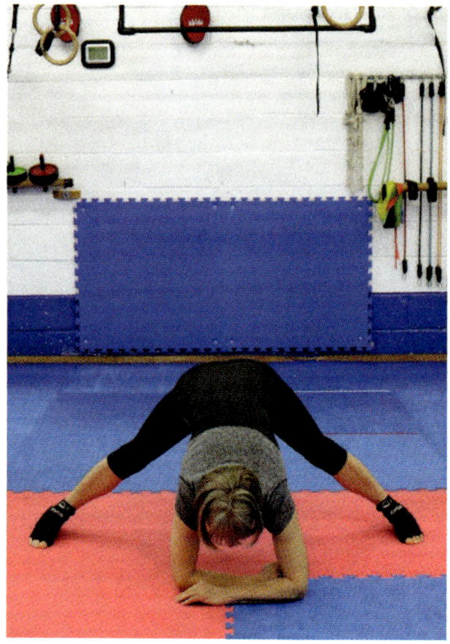

Figure 51

To loosen up and stretch the hip flexors and hamstrings

- Pivot your legs to front splits, with your right leg in front of you and your left leg behind you, with your left knee on the floor. Keep your toes out straight behind you and rest on the ball of your left foot. Put your palms on the floor in front of you, keeping your arms straight, left arm forward and right one slightly back. Lower your left hip towards the floor, going as low as possible. Hold for 10-15 seconds ***(Figure 52).***
- Move your hands closer to your right foot ***(Figure 53)*** and, if you can, rest your elbows on the floor for an extra stretch. Hold for 10-15 seconds ***(Figure 54).***
- Then move your right hand over the right leg, keeping your left hand on the inside of your right leg. Move both hands forward, close to your right foot ***(Figure 55)*** and try lowering yourself onto your elbow. Hold for 10-15 seconds ***(Figure 56)***.
- Return to a central, wide squat position and put your hands on the floor, or elbows if possible. Hold for 10-15 seconds ***(Figures 57 & 58).***

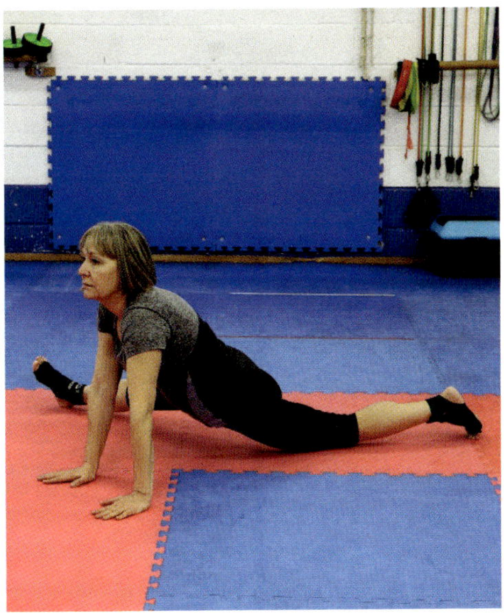

Figure 52

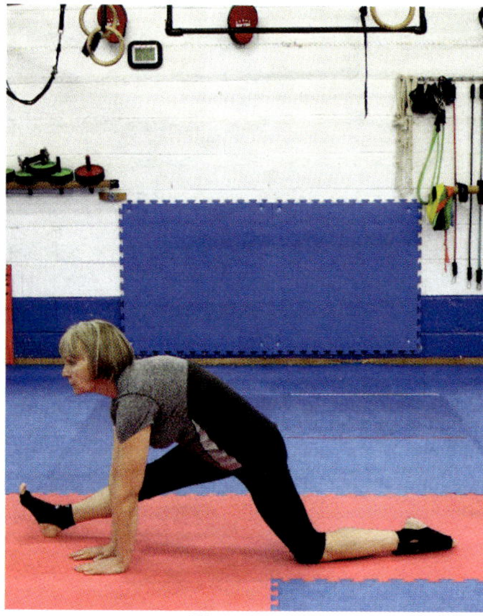

Figure 53

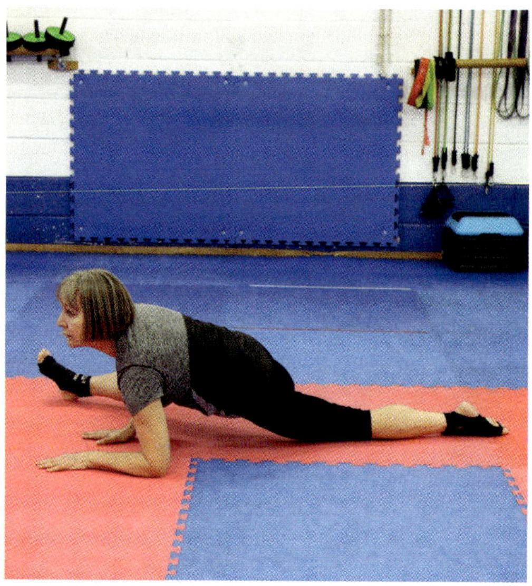

Figure 54

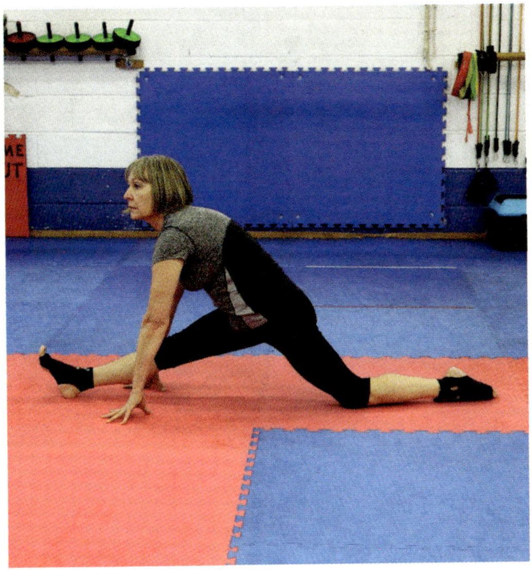

Figure 55

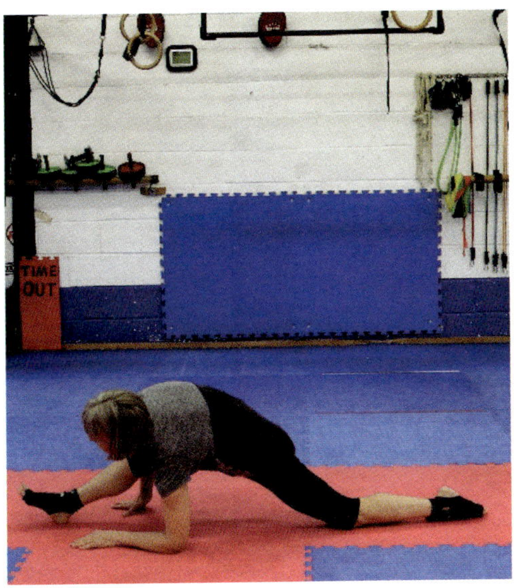

Figure 56

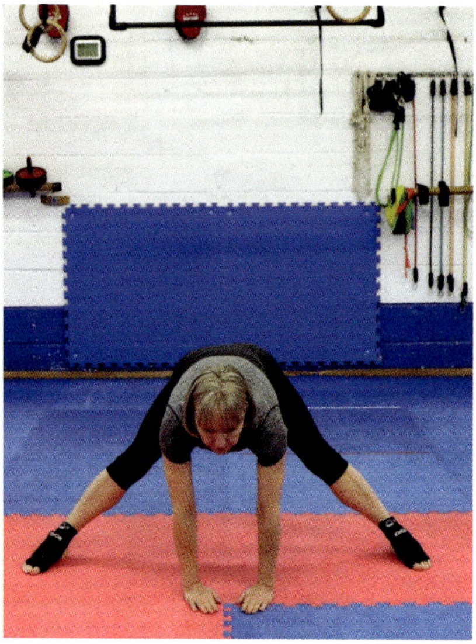

Figure 57

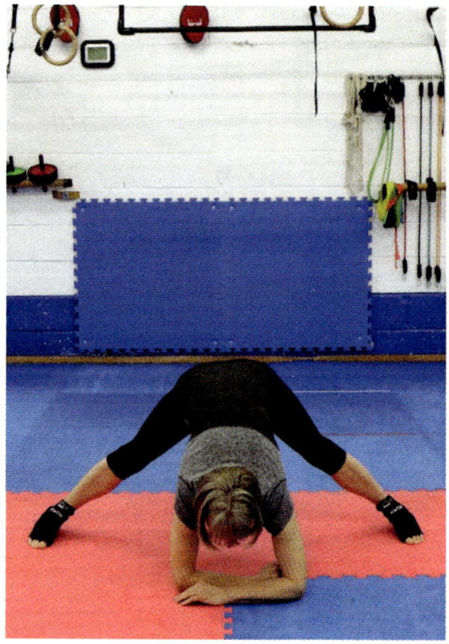

Figure 58

- Repeat the same stretch on the other side. Pivot your legs to right front splits, with your left leg in front of you and your right leg behind you, with your right knee on the floor. Keep your toes out straight behind you and rest on the ball of your right foot. Put your palms on the floor in front of you, keeping your arms straight, right arm forward and left one slightly back. Lower your right hip towards the floor, going as low as possible. Hold for 10-15 seconds ***(Figure 59).***
- Move your hands closer to your left foot ***(Figure 60)*** and, if you can, rest your elbows on the floor for an extra stretch. Hold for 10-15 seconds ***(Figure 61).***
- Then move your left hand over your left leg, keeping your right hand on the inside of your left leg. Move both hands forward, close to your left foot ***(Figure 62)*** and try lowering yourself onto your elbow. Hold for 10-15 seconds ***(Figure 63)***.
- Return to the centre position, widen your legs to your maximum comfortable stretch and rest your palms or elbows on the floor again ***(Figures 64 & 65)***.

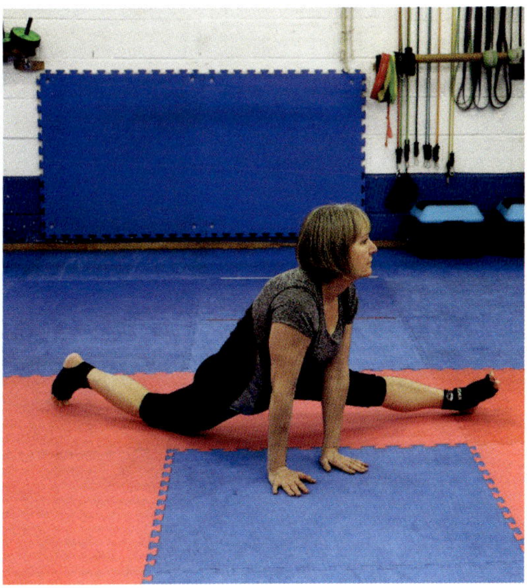

Figure 59

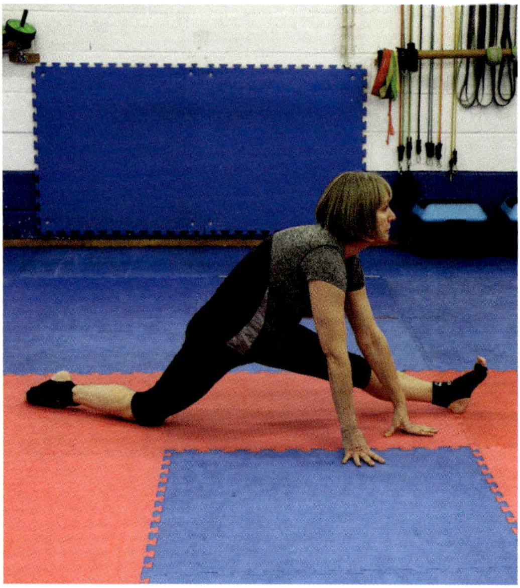

Figure 60

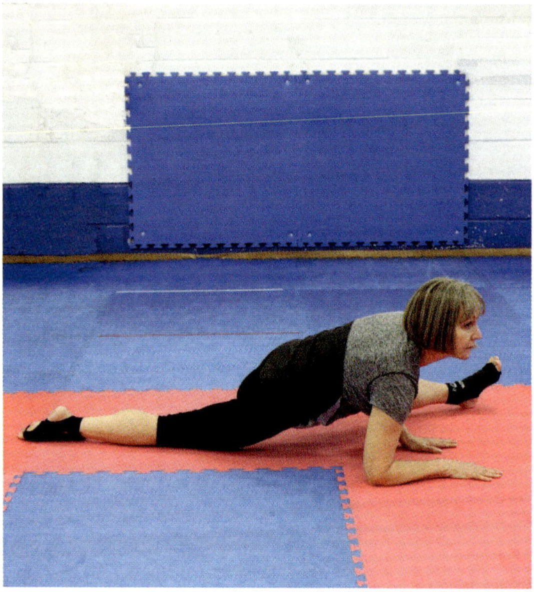

Figure 61

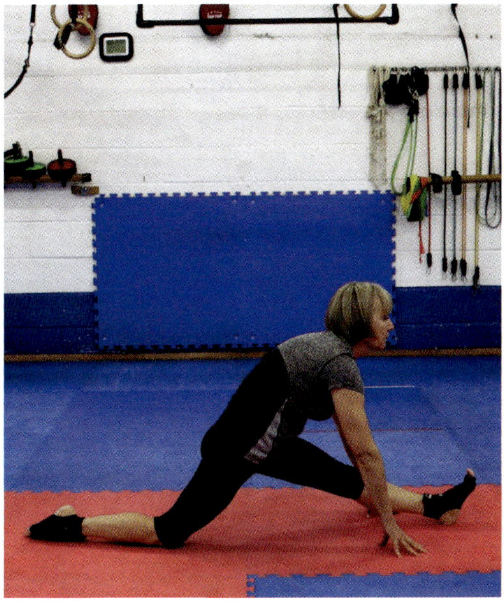

Figure 62

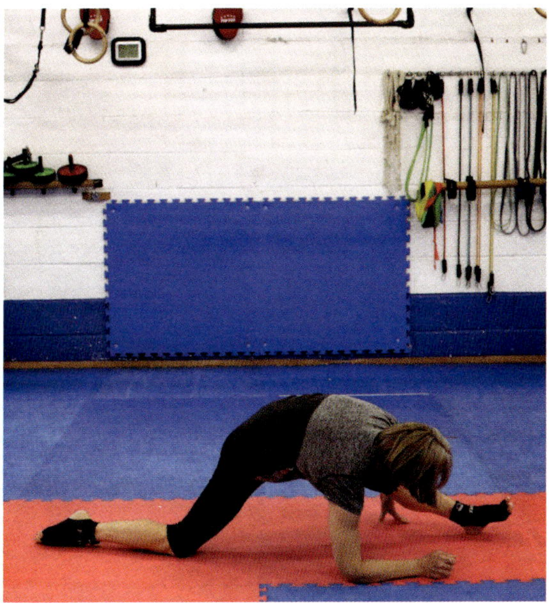

Figure 63

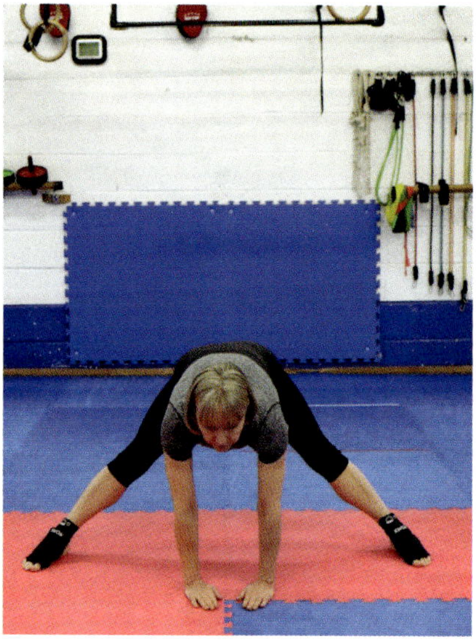

Figure 64

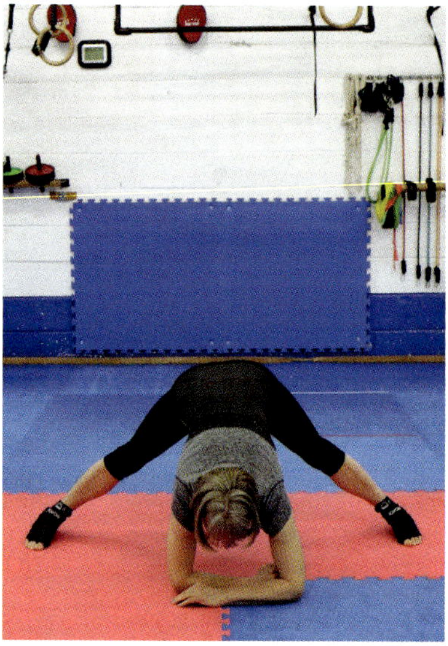

Figure 65

To loosen up and stretch the hip flexors and hamstrings

- Step forward with your left leg and bend your left knee to 90 degrees. Raise your left hand up and, with your right hand, reach your right foot and pull it up to your right glutes. Hold for 10-15 seconds ***(Figure 66).***
- Repeat the same to the other side. Hold for 10-15 seconds ***(Figure 67).***

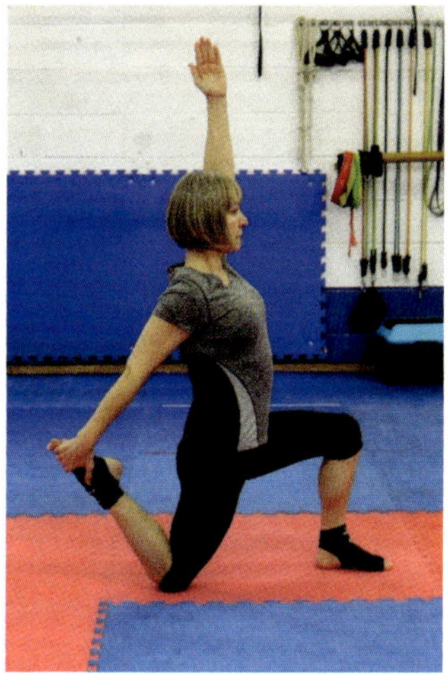

Figure 66

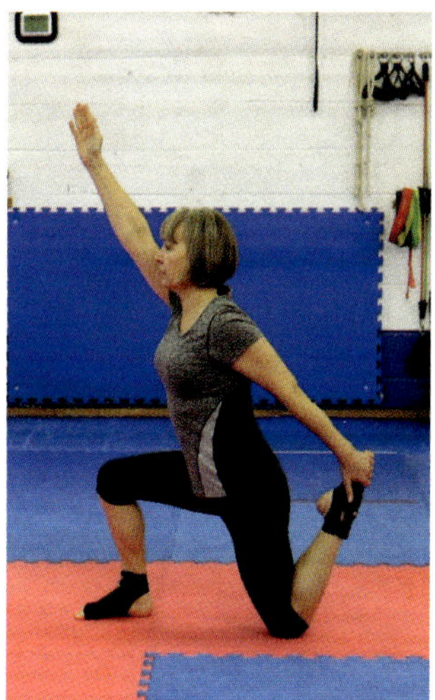

Figure 67

- Put your left foot down, raise your left knee and stretch the leg out behind you, resting on the toes. Move to the yoga '*warrior*' position by leaning your body at a 45-degree angle over your right leg. Stretch your hands up parallel with your head Hold this position for 10-15 seconds ***(Figure 68).*** Then raise your body to a vertical posture '*upper warrior*' yoga position with hands up. Hold for another 10-15 seconds ***(Figure 69).***

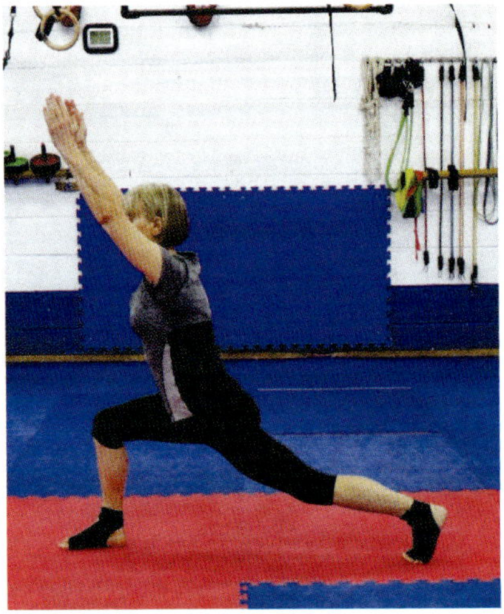

Figure 68

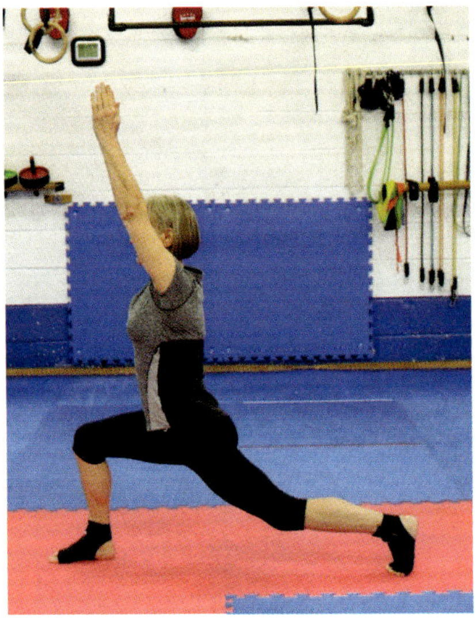

Figure 69

- Move your weight over to your right leg, lower your body down as far as you can and squat over your right leg. Stretch your left leg out, resting your left heel on the floor, toes pointing up. Keeping the right foot fully on the floor, stretch your hands out in front of you ***(Figure 70)***. If you find it difficult to have your right foot fully on the floor, you can lift the heel up slightly, and you can rest your hands on the floor, right hand inside your left leg and left hand on the other side of the left leg. Hold this stretch for 10-15 seconds ***(Figure 71)***.

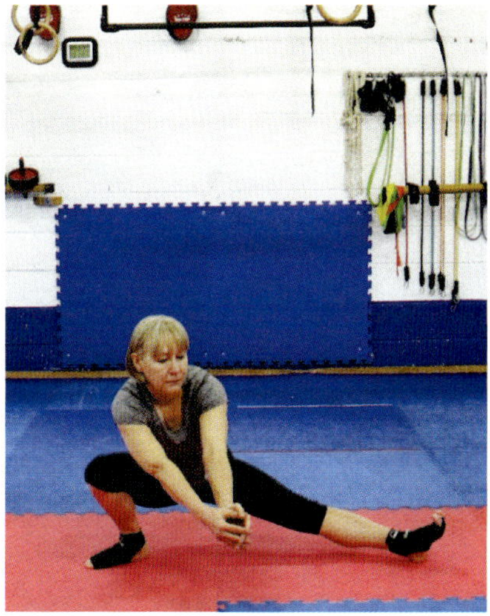

Figure 70

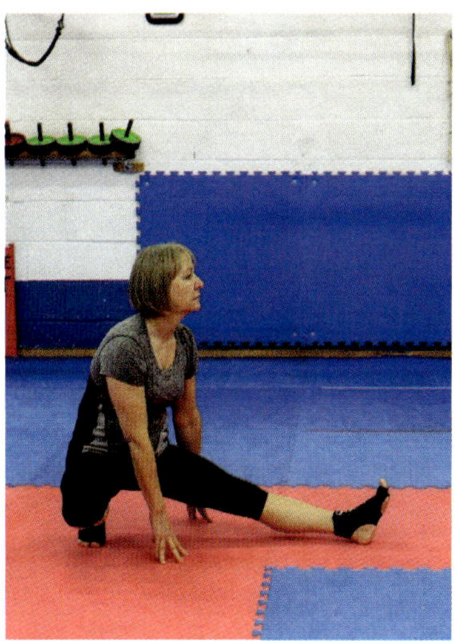

Figure 71

- Repeat the same stretch by moving to the other side and lowering your body down as far as possible to squat over to your left leg. Stretch your right leg out, resting your right heel on the floor, toes pointing up. Keeping the left foot fully on the floor, stretch your hands out in front of you ***(Figure 72)***. If you find it difficult to have your left foot fully on the floor, you can lift the heel up slightly, and you can rest your hands on the floor, left hand inside your right leg and right hand on the other side of the right leg. Hold this stretch for 10-15 seconds ***(Figure 73).***

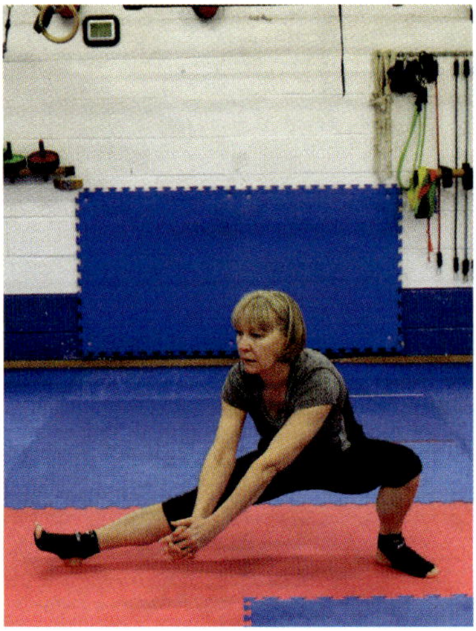

Figure 72

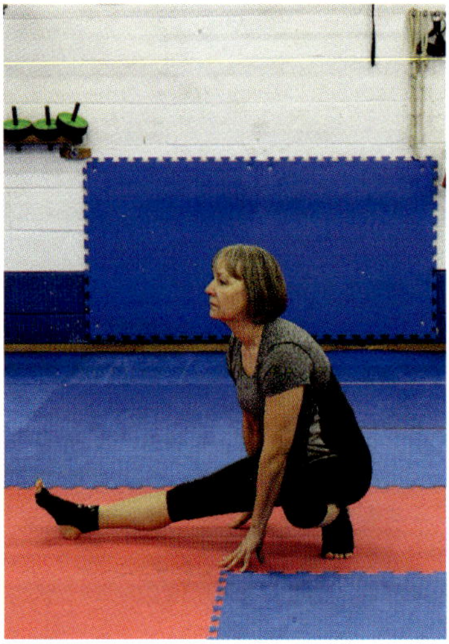

Figure 73

- Repeat the same stretch by moving and lowering your body to squat over your right leg. Stretch your left leg out, resting your left heel on the floor, toes pointing up. Keeping the right foot fully on the floor, stretch your hands out in front of you ***(Figure 74)***. If you find it difficult to have your right foot fully on the floor, you can lift your heel up slightly, and you can rest your hands on the floor, right hand inside your left leg and left hand on the other side of your left leg. Hold this stretch for 10-15 seconds ***(Figure 75)***.

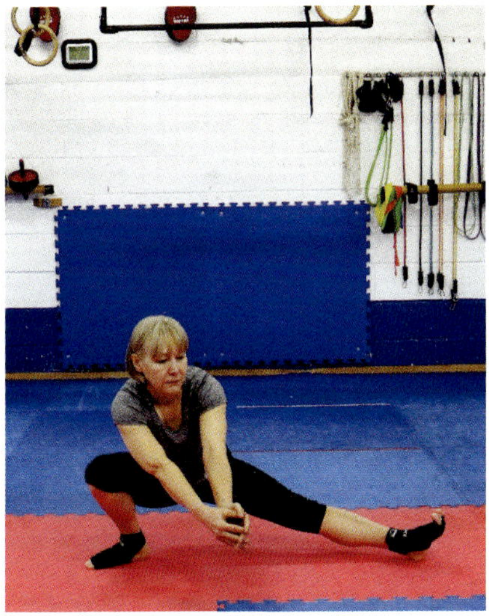

Figure 74

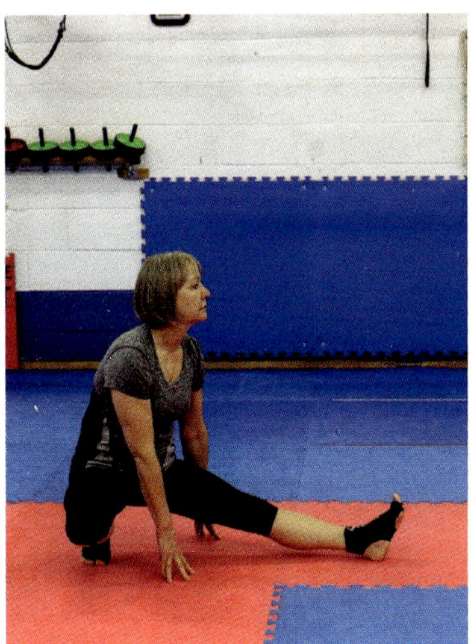

Figure 75

- Return to the yoga *warrior* position by leaning your body at a 45-degree angle, this time over your left leg with your right leg straight out behind you. Stretch your hands out parallel with your head (***Figure 76)***. Hold this position for 10-15 seconds and then raise your body to a vertical posture *upper warrior* position with hands up. Hold for another 10-15 seconds ***(Figure 77).***

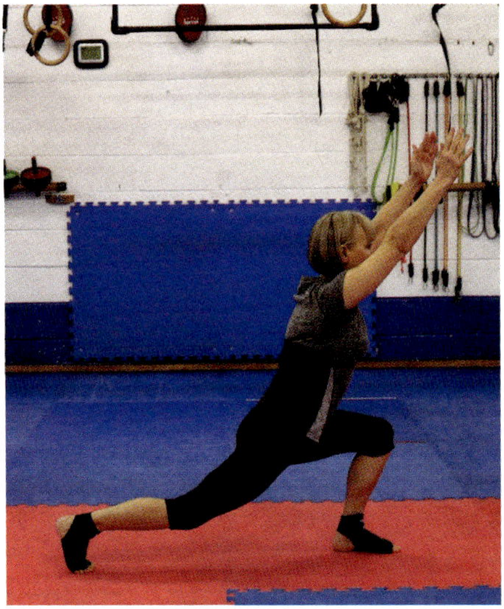

Figure 76

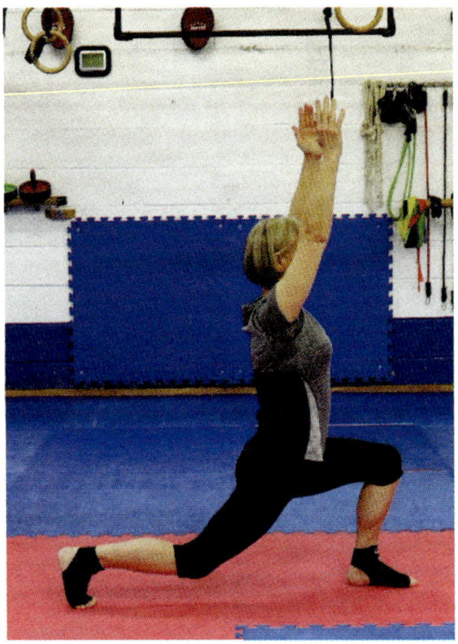

Figure 77

- Move your weight over to your left leg, lower your body and squat over your left leg. Stretch your right leg out, resting your right heel on the floor, toes pointing up. Keeping the left foot fully on the floor, stretch your hands out in front of you ***(Figure 78)***. If you find it difficult to have your left foot fully on the floor, you can lift the heel up slightly, and you can rest your hands on the floor, left hand inside your right leg and right hand on the other side of the right leg. Hold this stretch for 10-15 seconds ***(Figure 79).***

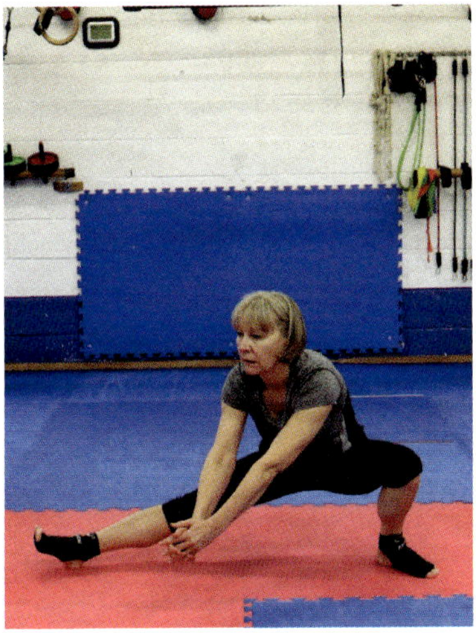

Figure 78

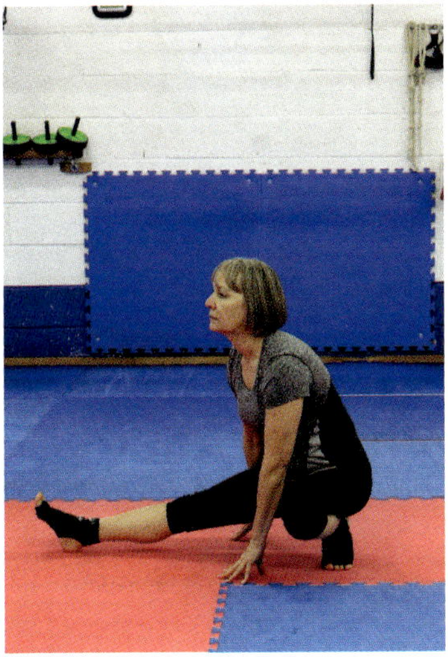

Figure 79

- Repeat the same stretch by moving to the other side and lowering your body to squat over to your right leg. Stretch your left leg out, resting your left heel on the floor, toes pointing up. Keeping the right foot fully on the floor, stretch your hands out in front of you ***(Figure 80)***. If you find it difficult to have your right foot fully on the floor, you can lift the heel up slightly, and you can rest your hands on the floor, right hand inside your left leg and left hand on the other side of left leg. Hold this stretch for 10-15 seconds ***(Figure 81).***

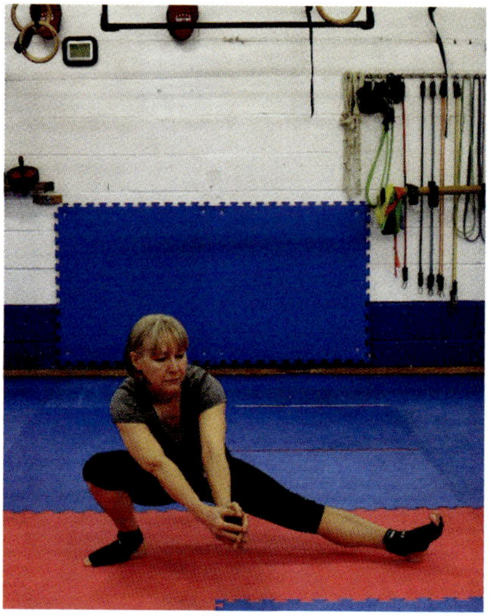

Figure 80

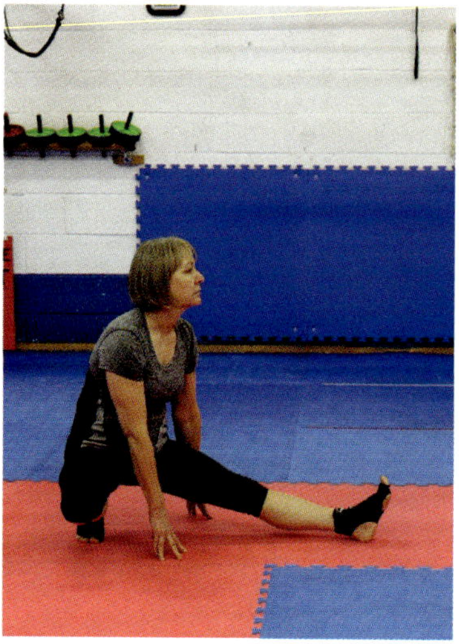

Figure 81

- Repeat the same stretch by moving and lowering your body to squat over your left leg. Stretch your right leg out, resting your right heel on the floor, toes pointing up. Keeping the left foot fully on the floor, stretch your hands out in front of you ***(Figure 82)***. If you find it difficult to have your left foot fully on the floor, you can lift the heel up slightly, and you can rest your hands on the floor, left hand inside your right leg and right hand on the other side of your right leg. Hold this stretch for 10-15 seconds ***(Figure 83)***.

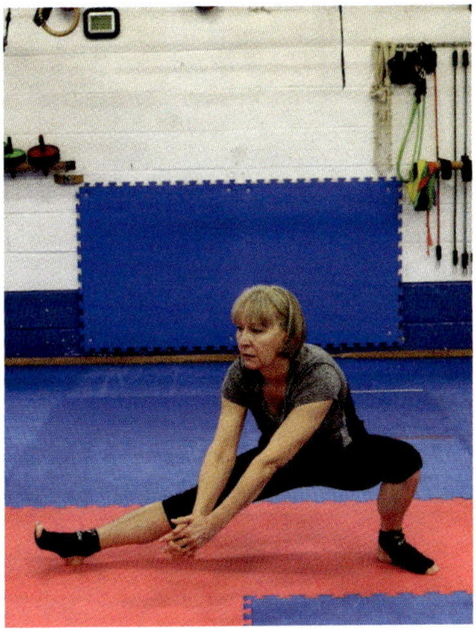

Figure 82

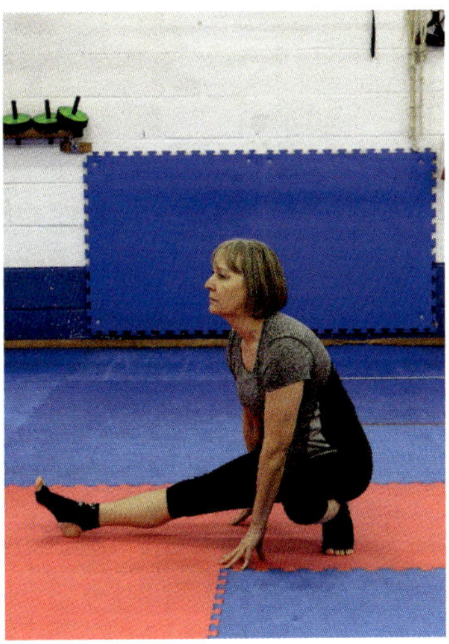

Figure 83

- Following these exercises move to a comfortable central box splits position, hands relaxed on the floor ***(Figure 84).***
- Put both legs together in a squat position and put your palms on your knees ***(Figure 85 side view)***. Gently elevate yourself to a standing position. Shake your arms and legs to loosen up.

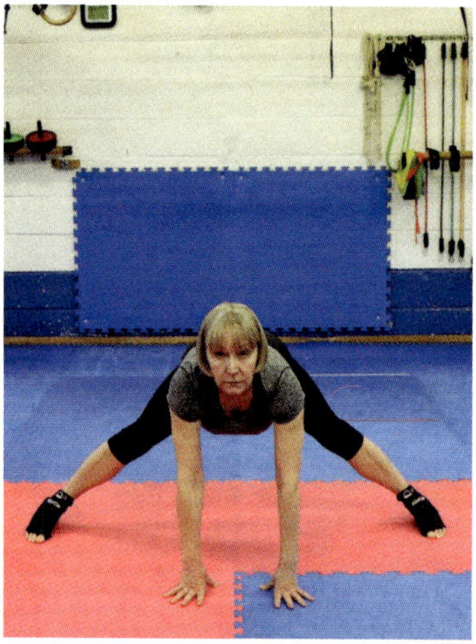

Figure 84

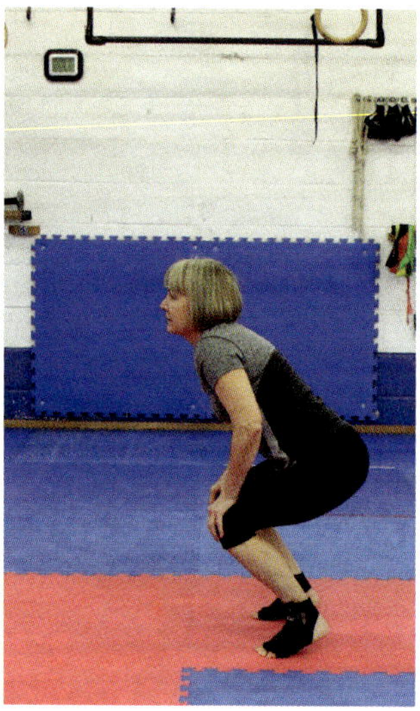

Figure 85 (side view)

Rest for 30 seconds with a light drink of water before moving on.

Workout exercise sets

Do all the following exercises for *1 minute each.*

Repeat each set of exercises twice at Beginner level (from week 1 to week 12). Increase repetition to three times each set of exercises after week 12.

All exercises should be done at a speed with which you are comfortable.

EXERCISE SET 1

1 minute - Wide leg low squats

- From a standing position, open your feet wider than your hips, turn your toes slightly out and lift your heels off the floor. Stretch your hands out at shoulder level in front of you ***(Figure 86),*** lower your hips and squat to knee level, keeping your body as vertical as you can with shoulders back and chin up.
- Move forward in four gentle hops, lowering yourself as you move until the squat is at knee level ***(always keep your knees over your toes as you squat) (Figure 87)***. Then reverse the move by gently hopping backwards until you are back at the high squat position ***(Figure 86)***.
- Breathe in on the way down, breathe out on the way up and gently push hips forward when standing up.
- Repeat the full sequence for one minute.

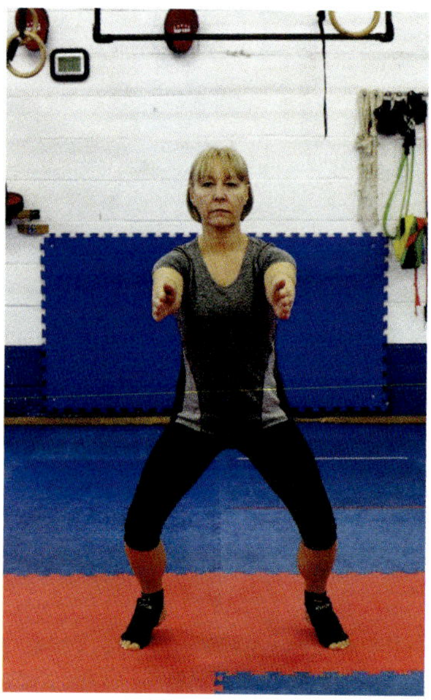

Figure 86

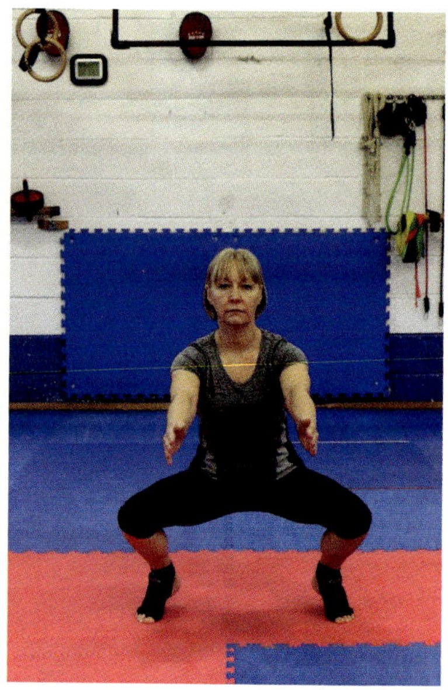

Figure 87

1 minute - High plank running squats

- Go to the high plank position: arms straight, palms on the floor shoulder-width apart, feet about 25cm apart and resting on the balls of your feet ***(Figure 88 side view).***
- With your right leg straight out behind you, in running motion, bring the left leg forward between your arms with knee low to the floor ***(Figure 89 side view).***
- Alternately switch the legs in a running motion, keeping knees low to the floor at all times ***(Figure 90 side view)***.
- Repeat full sequence for one minute.

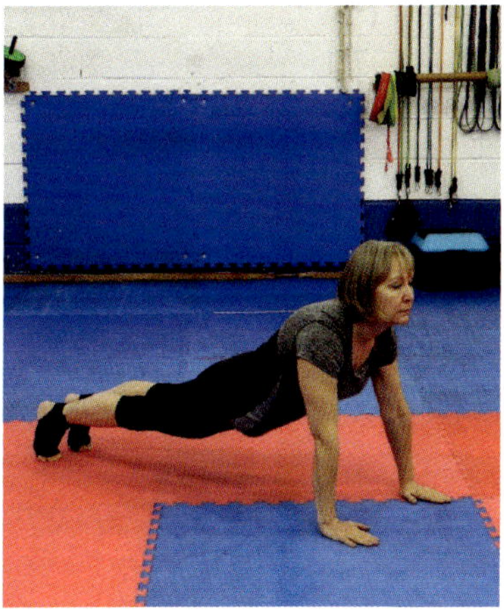

Figure 88 (side view)

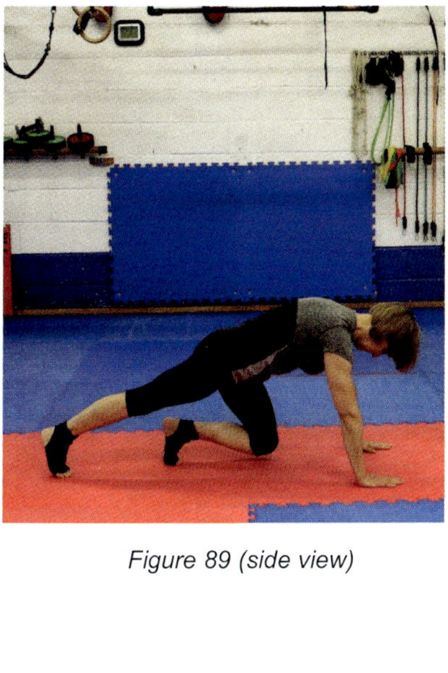

Figure 89 (side view)

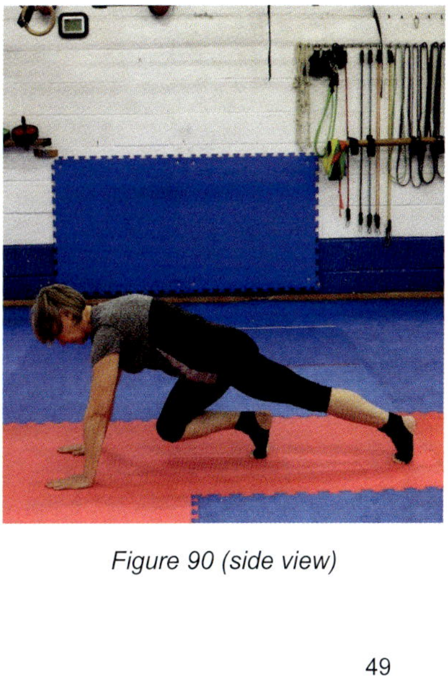

Figure 90 (side view)

1 minute - Short jump lunges

- From a standing position, open your feet to shoulder width apart with arms relaxed down on the side of your body ***(Figure 91)***.
- In gentle jumping mode, move your left leg forward and your right leg back, lowering your right knee to the floor by your left heel. At the same time, raise your hands high above your head ***(Figure 92 side view)*** and then return to standing position ***(Figure 93)***.
- Repeat with the other leg, moving your right leg forward and your left leg back by lowering your left knee to the floor by your right heel. Raise your hands high above your head ***(Figure 94 side view)*** and then return to standing position.
- Repeat full sequence for one minute.

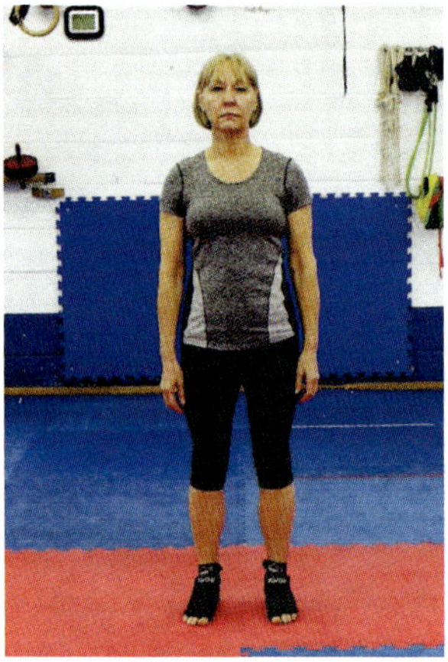

Figure 91

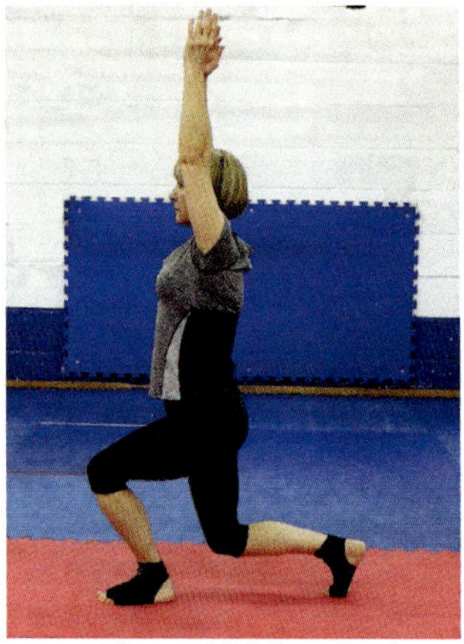

Figure 92 (side view)

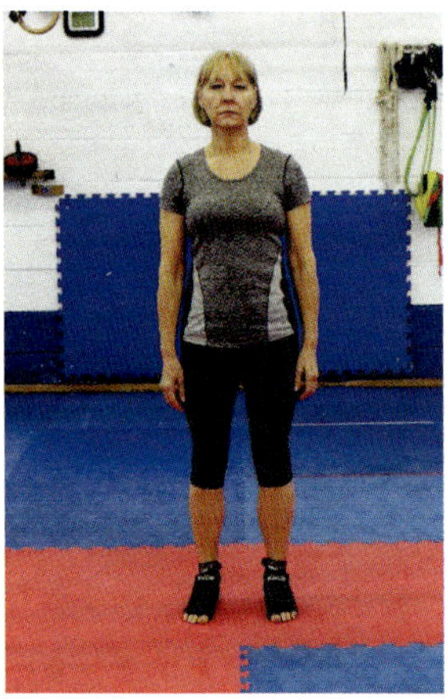

Figure 93

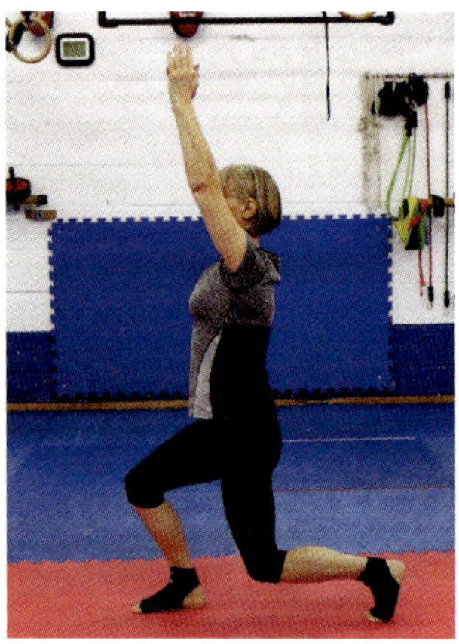

Figure 94 (side view)

Rest for 30 seconds before continuing.

EXERCISE SET 2

1 minute - Macedonian heavy dance squats

- In a standing position, have your hands close to your chest and open your feet to no more than 25cm apart ***(Figure 95).***
- Squat down to a depth you are comfortable with, breathing in as you go, and extend your hands straight out at shoulder height, keeping both feet on the floor ***(Figure 96 side view).***
- On your out breath, return to a standing position, slowly elevate your right knee ***(Figure 97 side view)*** and extend your leg out in front of you ***(Figure 98 side view).***
- Return to standing position ***(Figure 99)*** and repeat the squat again ***(Figure 100 side view).*** This time on your out breath, return to a standing position, slowly elevate your left knee ***(Figure 101 side view)*** and extend your left leg out in front of you ***(Figure 102 side view).***
- Repeat full sequence for one minute.

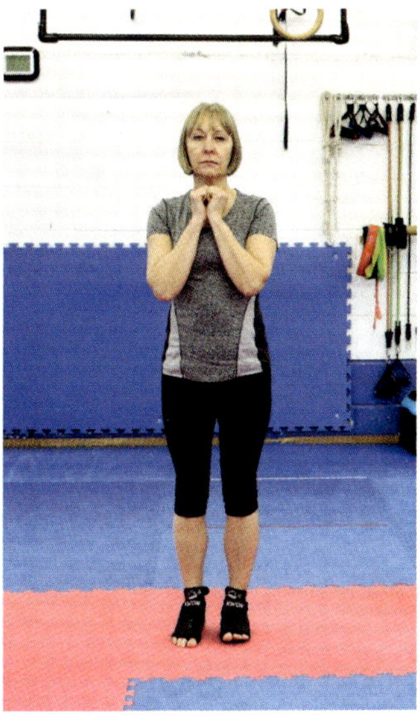

Figure 95

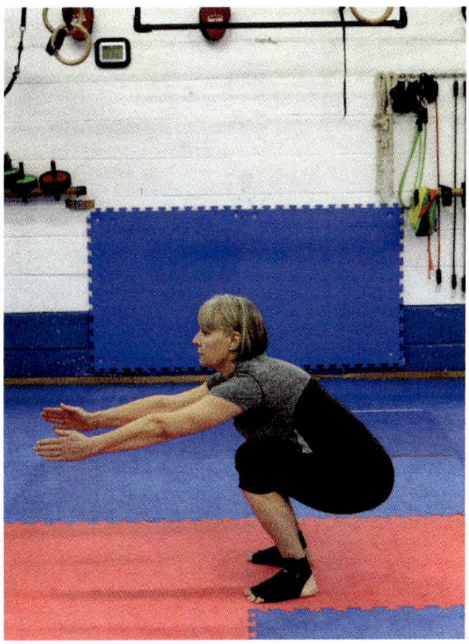

Figure 96 (side view)

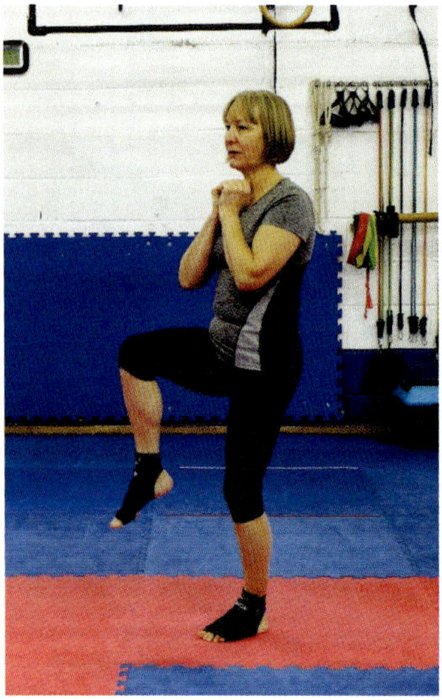

Figure 97 (side view)

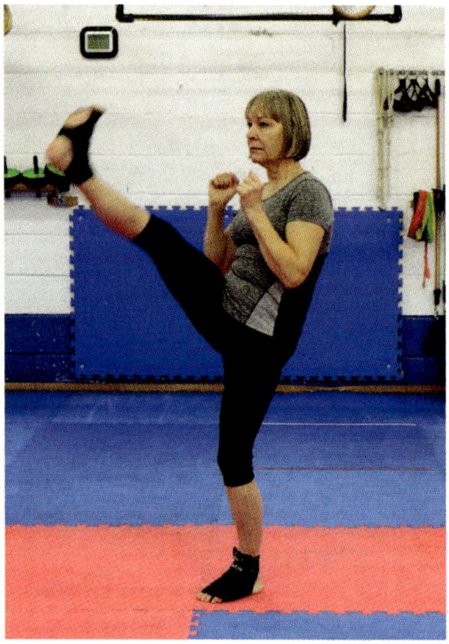

Figure 98 (side view)

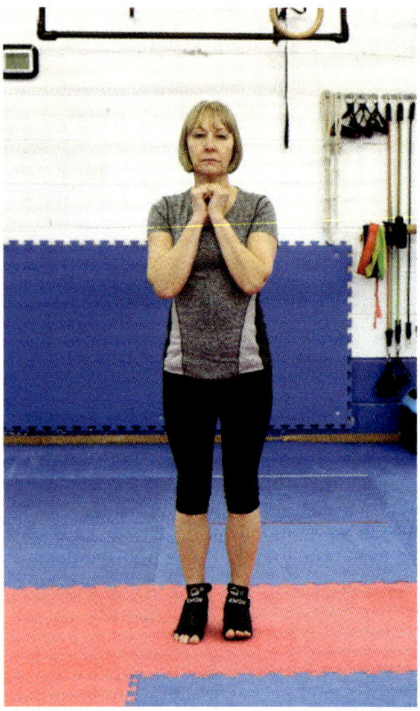

Figure 99

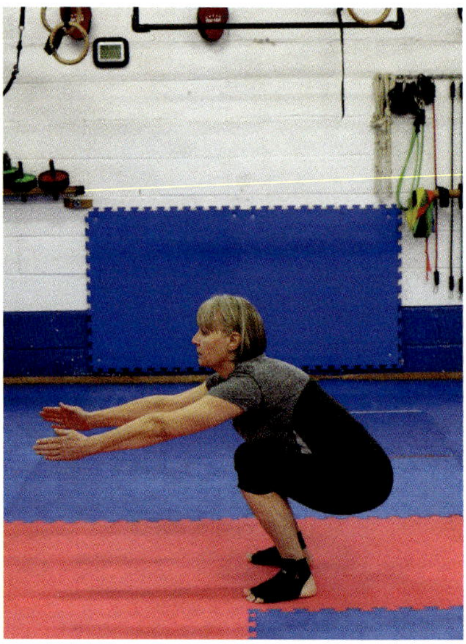

Figure 100 (side view)

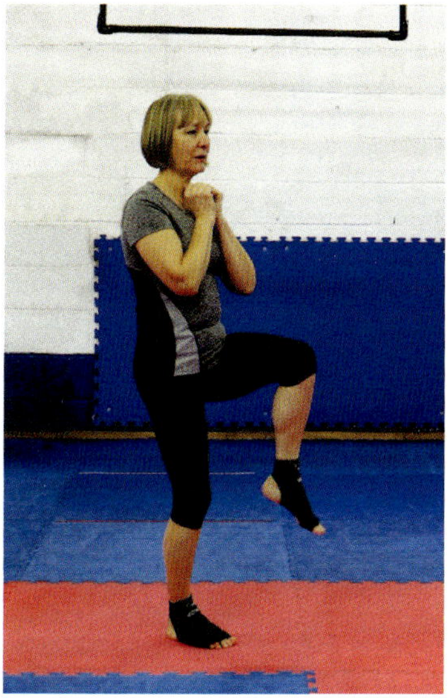

Figure 101 (side view)

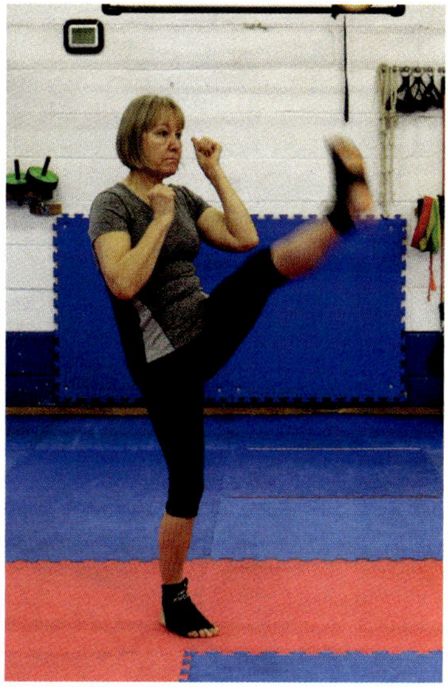

Figure 102 (side view)

1 minute - Basketball jumps

- In a standing position, open your feet no more than 25cm apart and raise your heels up off the floor ***(Figure 103)***.
- Drop down to a squat position until your heels touch your glutes, keeping your heels off the floor, breathe out and touch the floor with your hands ***(Figure 104).***
- Keeping your feet parallel, gently jump up in the air, raising your hands high above your head and breathing in ***(Figure 105).*** Then drop down to a squat position until your heels touch your glutes again, keeping your heels off the floor, breathing out and touching the floor with your hands ***(Figure 106).***
- Repeat full sequence for one minute.

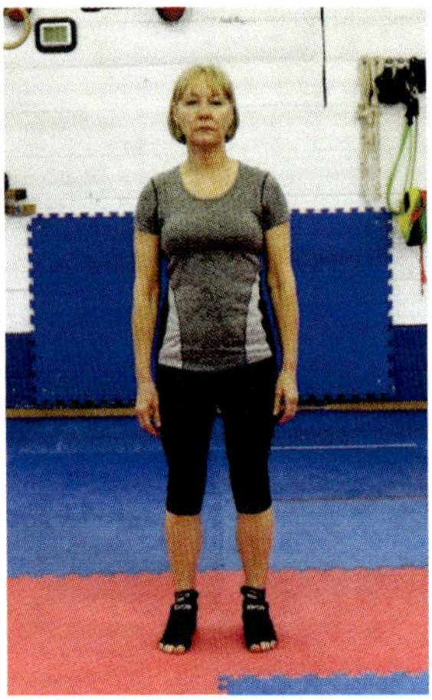

Figure 103

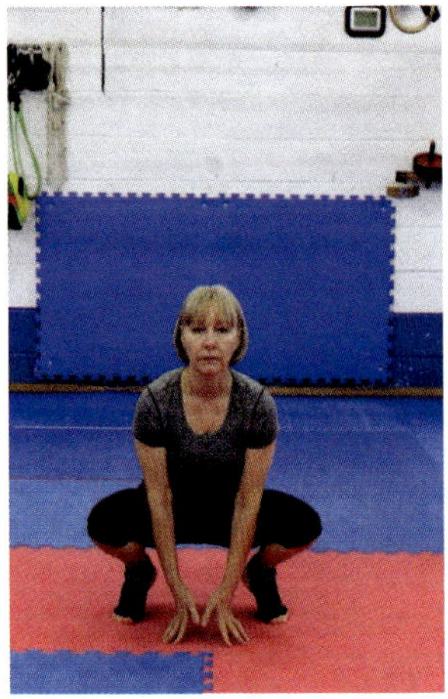

Figure 104

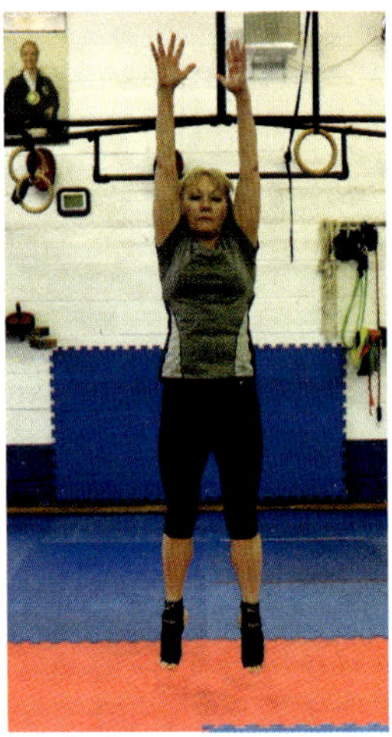

Figure 105

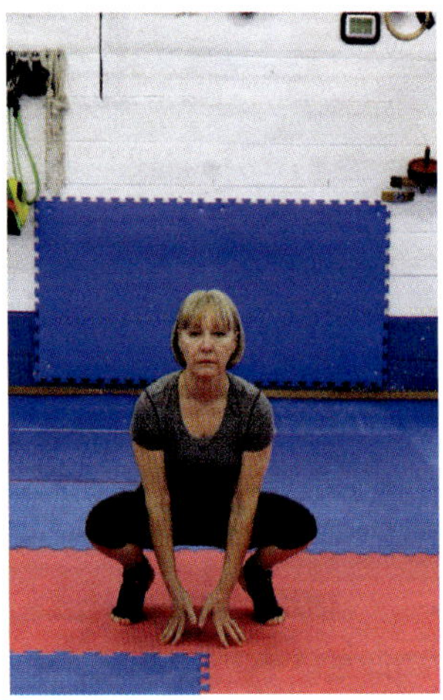

Figure106

1 minute - <u>High plank wide squats with heels on the floor</u>

- Go to the high plank position: arms straight, palms on the floor shoulder-width apart, feet about 25cm apart ***(Figure 107 side view)***.
- Jump to full squat position with both legs forward, landing softly on the soles of your feet, with both feet flat on the floor, and cross your hands on your chest ***(Figure 108)***.
- Repeat full sequence for one minute.

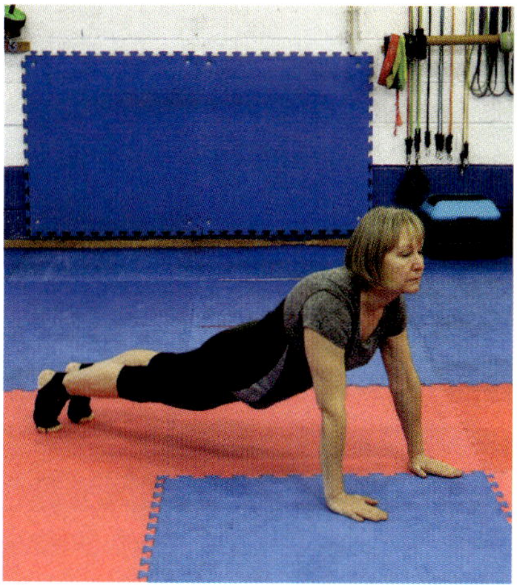

Figure 107 *(side view)*

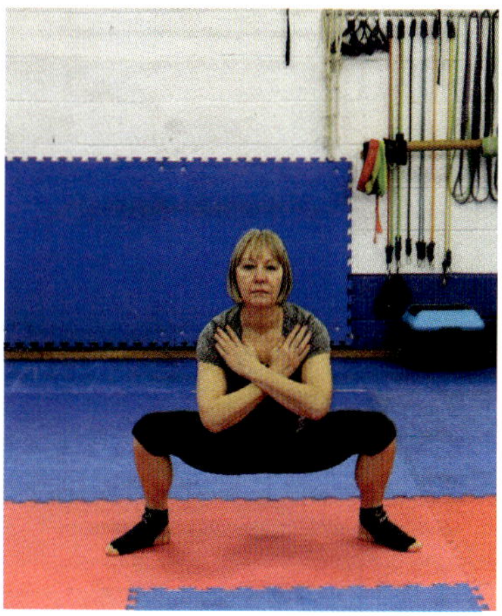

Figure 108

Rest for 30 seconds before continuing

EXERCISE SET 3

1 minute - Ski squats

- From a standing position with both feet together, raise your heels up and put your hands under your chin ***(Figure 109).***
- Keeping both knees and feet together, gently hop to the right in an approximate 90-degree turn and squat down, moving your arms across your body in a skiing motion ***(as if you were holding ski poles)***, ***(Figure 110).***
- Then stand straight up again ***(Figure 111)*** and gently hop to the left, repeating the motion ***(Figure 112)***.
- Continue jumping, alternating from side to side, for one minute.

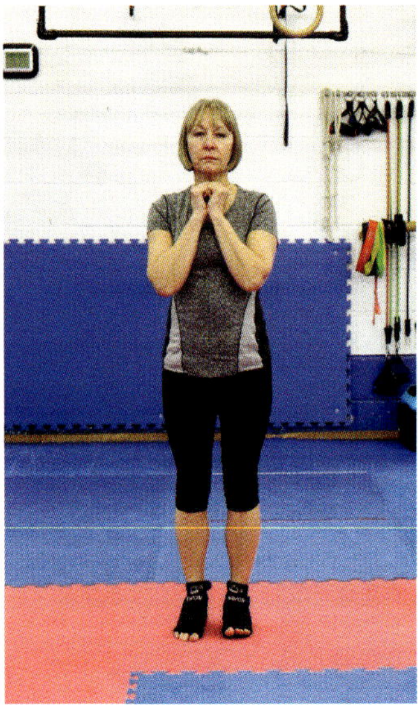

Figure 109

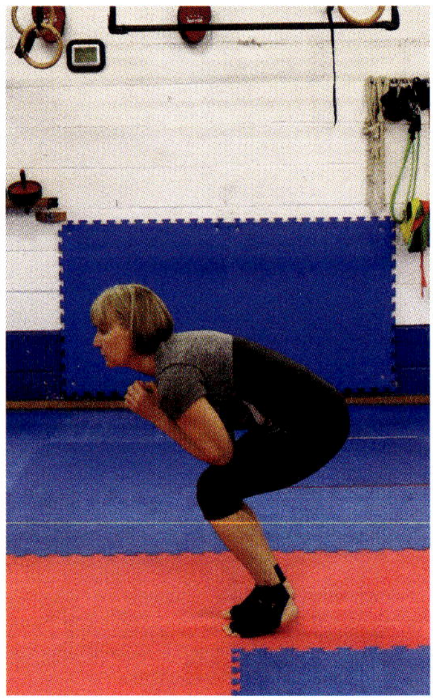

Figure 110

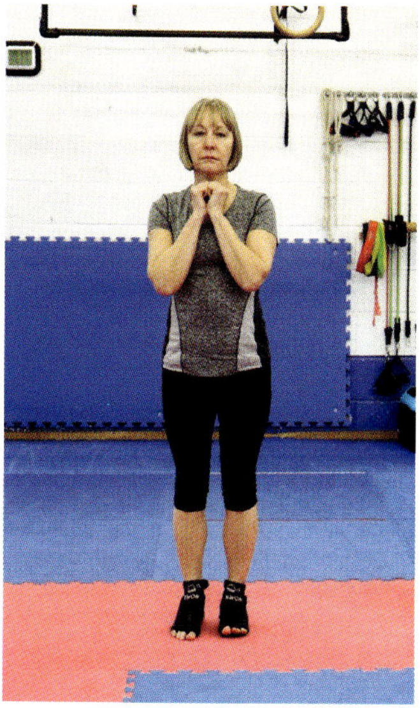

Figure 111

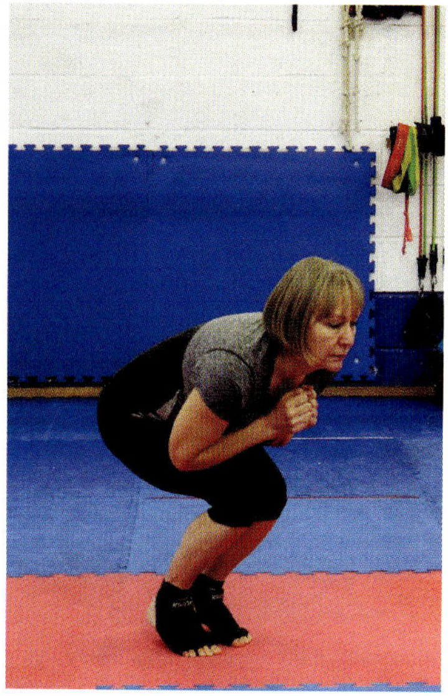

Figure 112

1 minute - Wide backward-stepping lunges

- In a standing position, open your feet to no more than 25cm apart. Rest both palms on your hips ***(Figure 113).***
- Move your left leg backwards to your maximum lunge position, stretching your arms straight up above your head ***(Figure 114 side view***).
- Return to left leg forward to standing position ***(Figure 115).***
- Move your right leg backwards to your maximum lunge position, stretching your arms straight up above your head ***(Figure 116 side view).***
- Repeat full sequence for one minute.

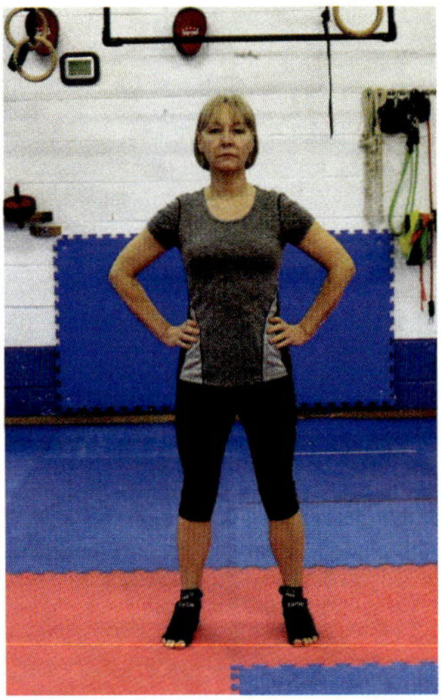

Figure 113

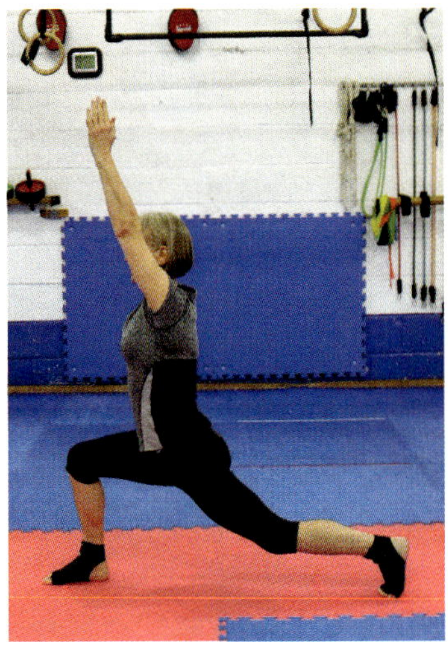

Figure 114 (side view)

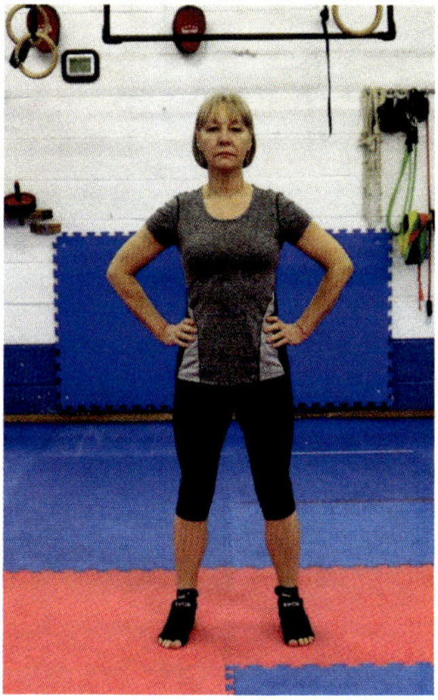

Figure 115

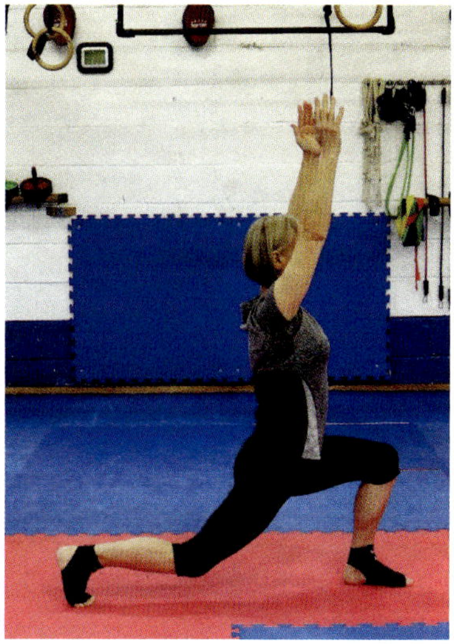

Figure 116 (side view)

1 minute - Cross-leg jumps with deep squats

- In a standing position ***(Figure 117),*** raise your heels up and jump-cross your legs, right leg over left leg, keeping your hands up in front of you ***(Figure 118).***
- Return to standing position ***(Figure 119),*** raise your heels up and now jump-cross your feet so that the left leg is over the right, keeping your hands up in front of you ***(Figure 120)***.
- Repeat full sequence ***(Figures 121-124)***.
- Lower yourself to a wide squat deep down with heels on the floor and touch the floor with your left hand, putting your palm on the floor if you can ***(Figure 125).***
- Elevate yourself slightly ***(Figure 126)*** and squat down deep again and touch the floor with your right hand, putting your palm on the floor if you can ***(Figure 127),*** then return to standing position ***(Figure 128)***.
- Repeat full sequence for one minute.

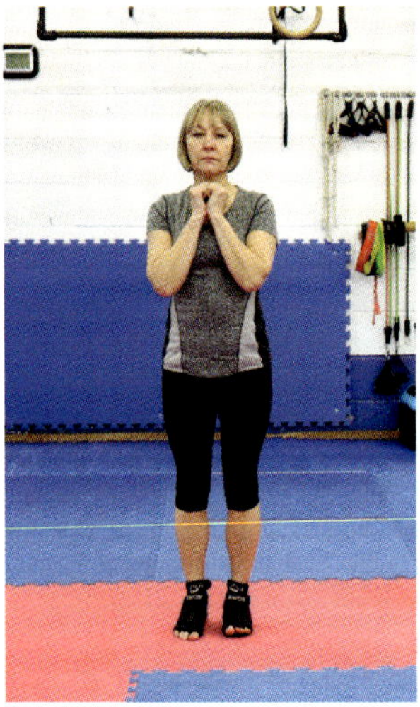

Figure 117

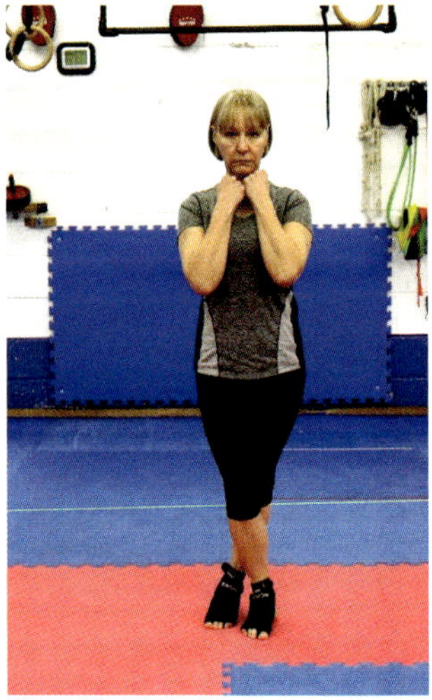

Figure 118

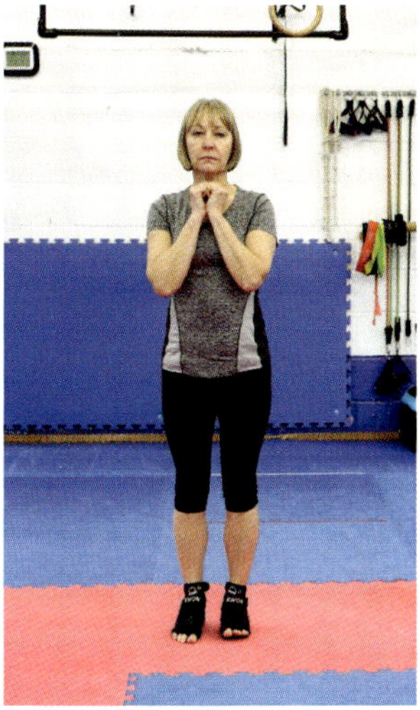

Figure 119

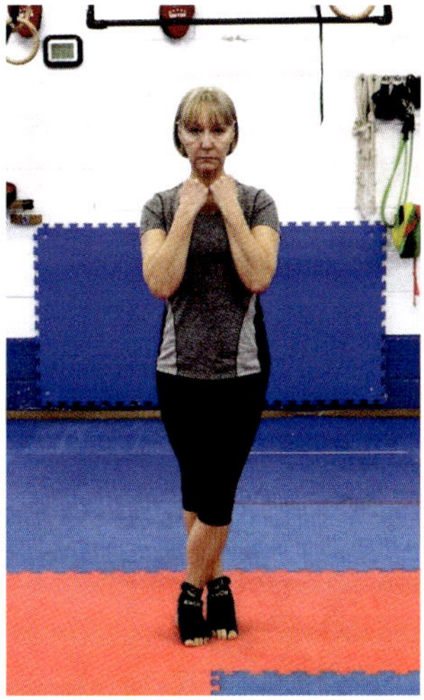

Figure120

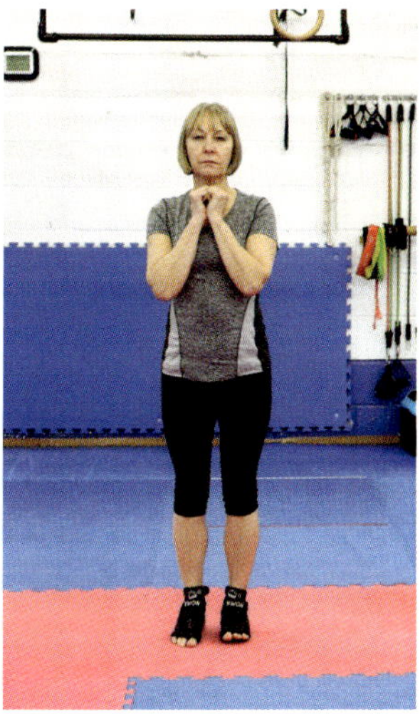

Figure 121

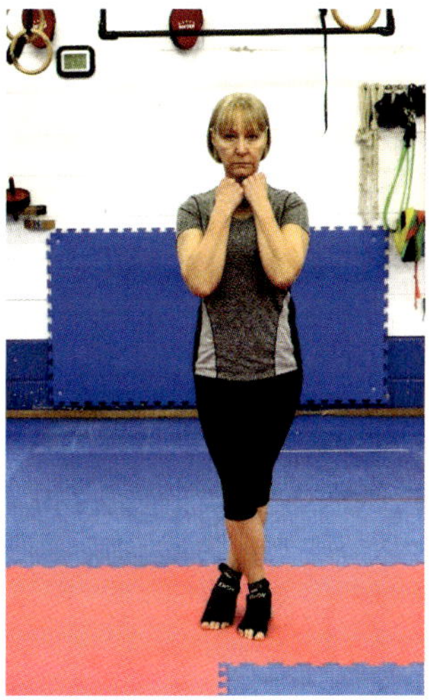

Figure 122

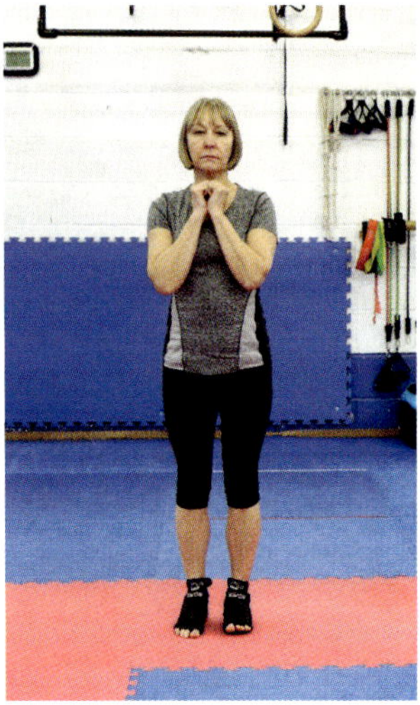

Figure 123

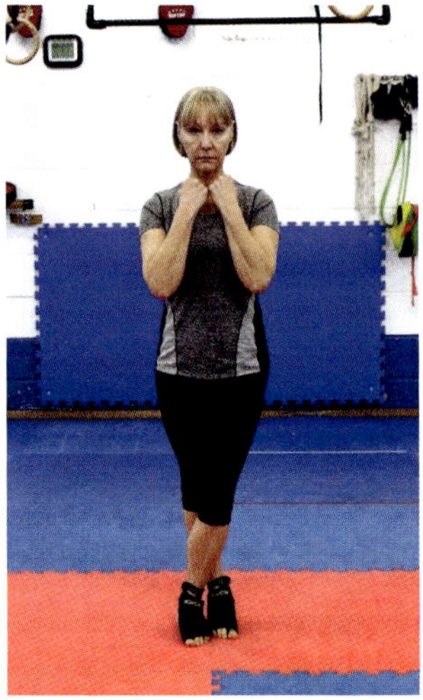

Figure124

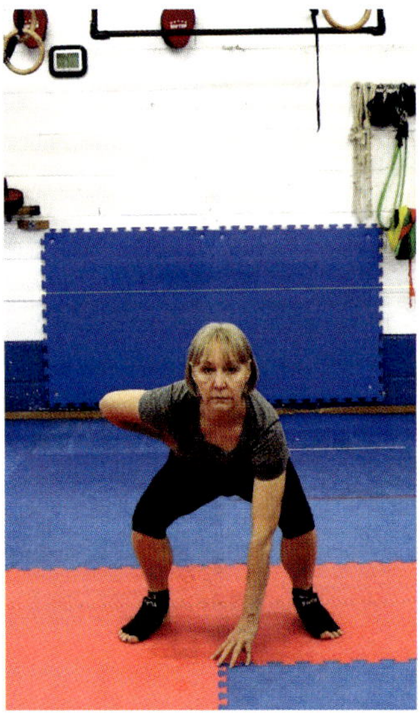

Figure 125

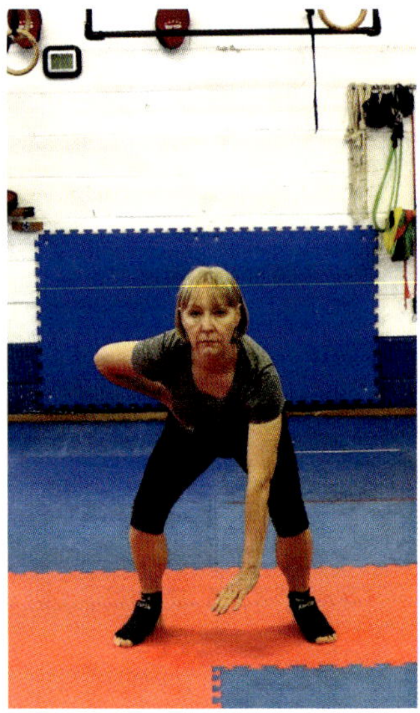

Figure 126

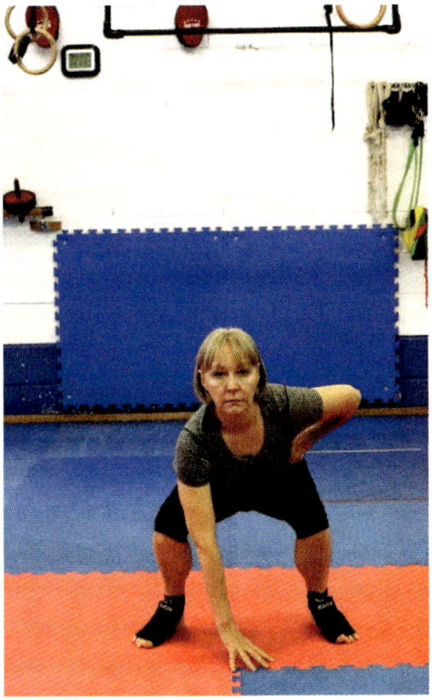

Figure 127

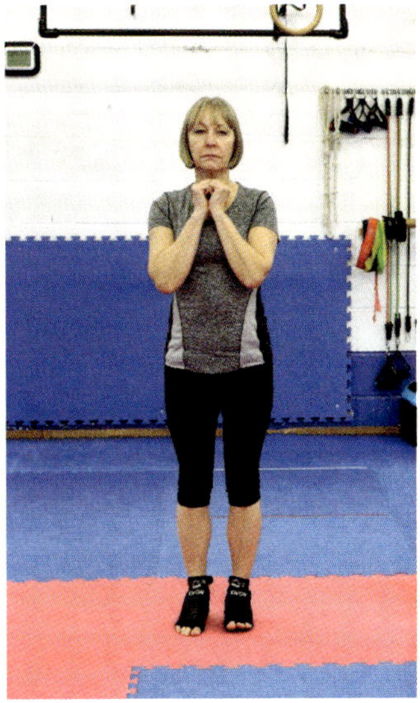

Figure 128

Rest for 30 seconds before continuing

Post-workout cool-down stretching

(This MUST be completed to relax the muscles)

- Lie down on your back with arms out in a cross position, legs together. Bend both knees up, bringing your feet close to your hips ***(Figure 129)***.
- Gently lower both legs down to the left side ***(Figure 130)*** then pull both knees up to your left elbow, keeping both shoulders on the floor with head turned to the right-hand side. Breathe out to relax and hold the position for 10-15 seconds ***(Figure 131)***.
- Extend ***(stretch)*** your left leg and grab the big toe of your left foot with your left hand, holding your leg straight out. With your right hand, grab the big toe and ball of your right foot and pull it behind you by first lowering your right shoulder towards the floor and then pulling and holding your bent right leg. Hold the stretch 10-15 seconds ***(Figure 132).***
- Move your legs back to the central position ***(Figure 133).***

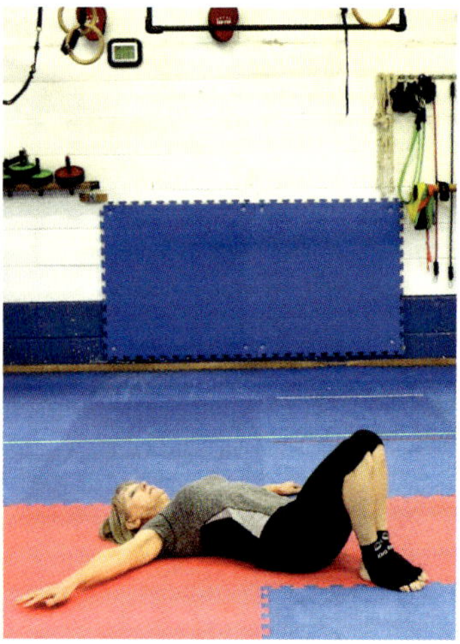

Figure 129

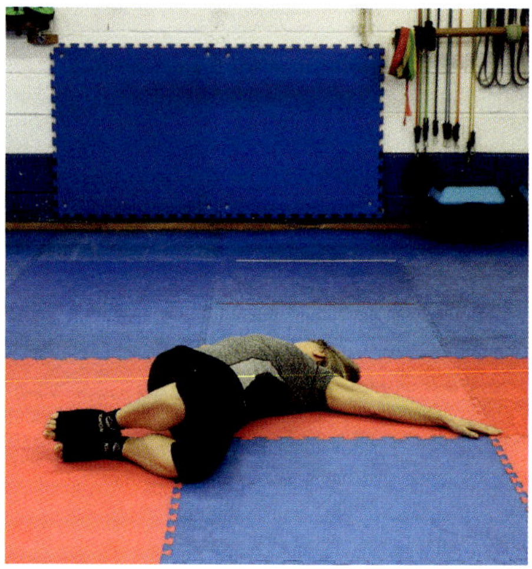

Figure 130

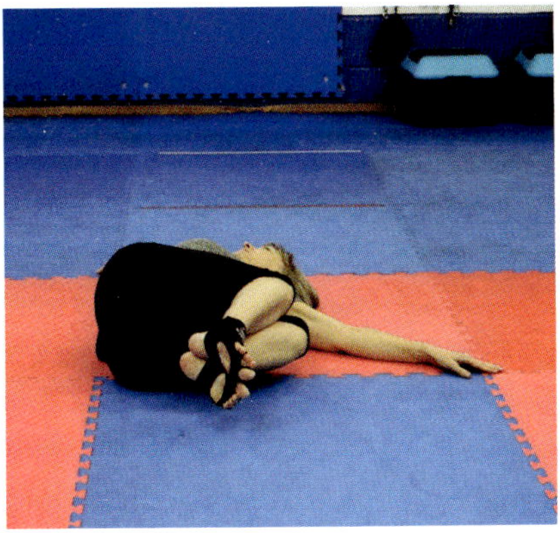

Figure 131

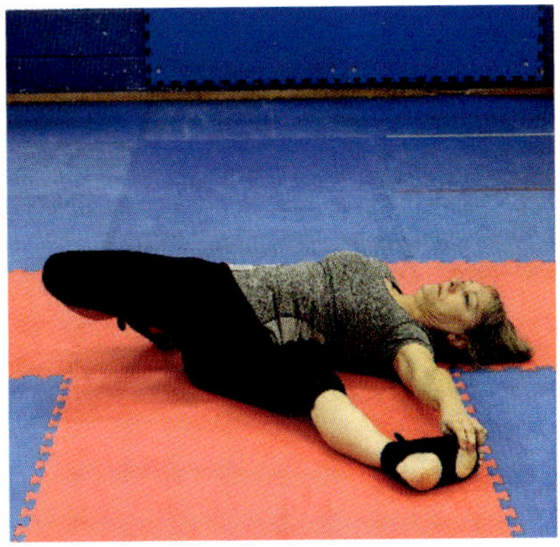

Figure 132

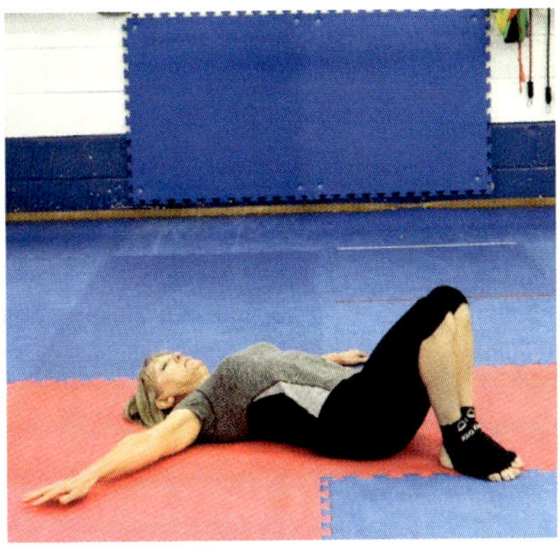

Figure 133

- Repeat the stretch sequence to the other side by lowering your bent legs to the right ***(Figure 134)***. Pull both knees up to your right elbow, keeping both shoulders on the floor and head turned to the left-hand side. Breathe out to relax and hold the position for 10-15 seconds ***(Figure 135)***.
- Extend ***(stretch)*** your right leg and grab the big toe of your right foot with your right hand, holding your leg straight out. With your left hand, grab the big toe and ball of your left foot and pull it behind you by first lowering your left shoulder towards the floor and then pulling and holding your bent left leg. Hold the stretch for 10-15 seconds (***Figure* 136).**
- Return to the starting position, legs together. Bend both knees up bringing your feet close to your hips (***Figure 137***).

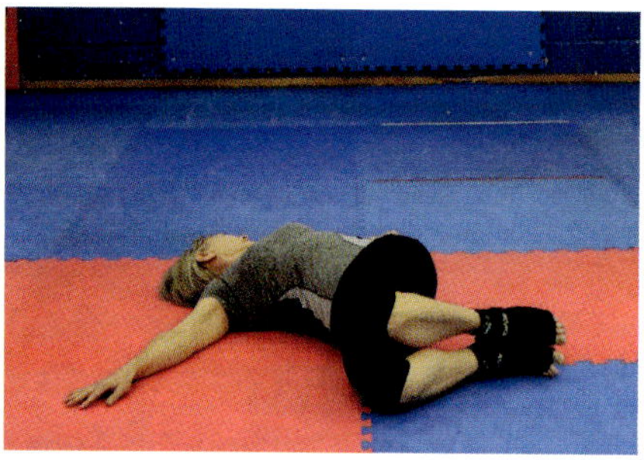

Figure 134

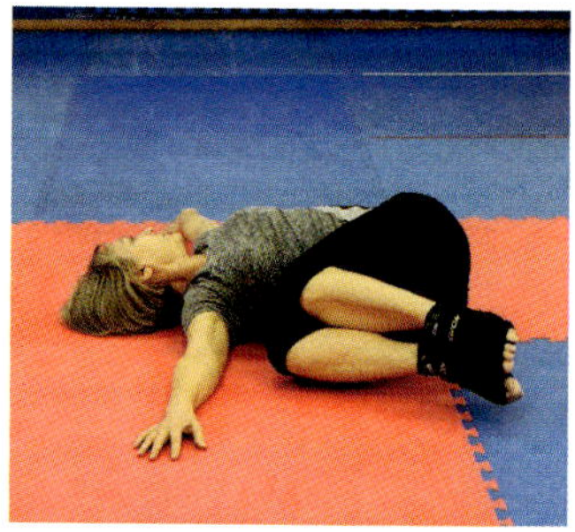

Figure 135

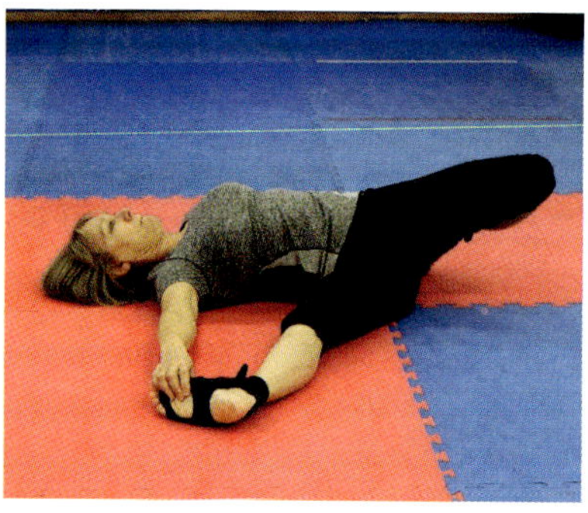

Figure 136

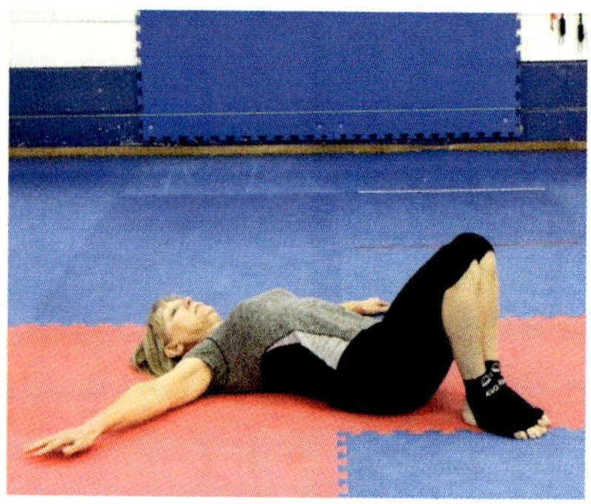

Figure 137

- Sit up with legs together, straight out in front of you. Gently lower your body down and try to touch your toes (use a belt or towel to help if you can't reach). Keep your chin up, breathe out and hold the stretch for 10-15 seconds ***(Figure 138)***.

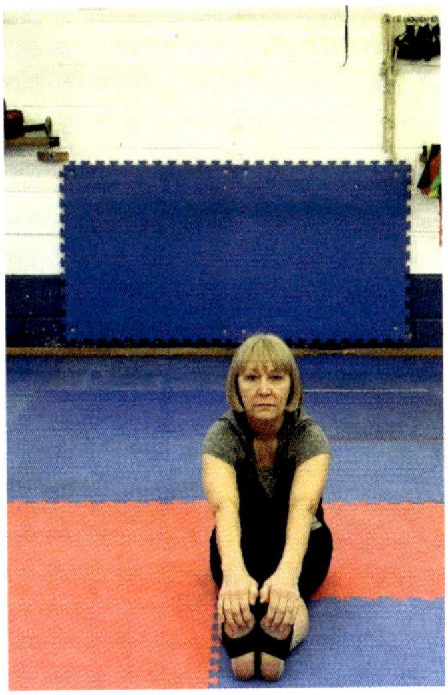

Figure 138

- Open your legs as wide as you can ***(Figure 139)*** and lower your body over your left leg. Reach your left foot with both hands, keeping your chin up ***(Figure 140)***. If you can't reach your left foot with your hands, use a rope or towel to help you ***(Figure 141)***. Breathe out and hold for 10-15 seconds.
- Keep hold of your foot with your right hand, move your left elbow to the inside of your left knee palm facing up, and gently twist your body to the right by pulling and bringing your head down towards your right knee ***(Figure 142).*** Breathe out and hold for 10-15 seconds. If you can't reach your left foot with your hand there are two alternate ways to do this stretch ***(Figures 143 & 144)***.

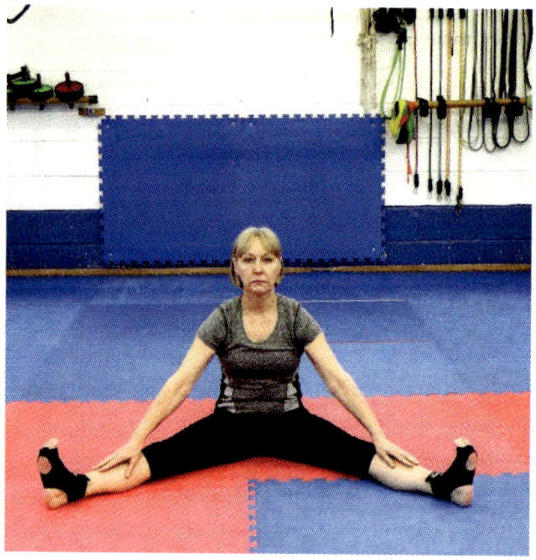

Figure 139

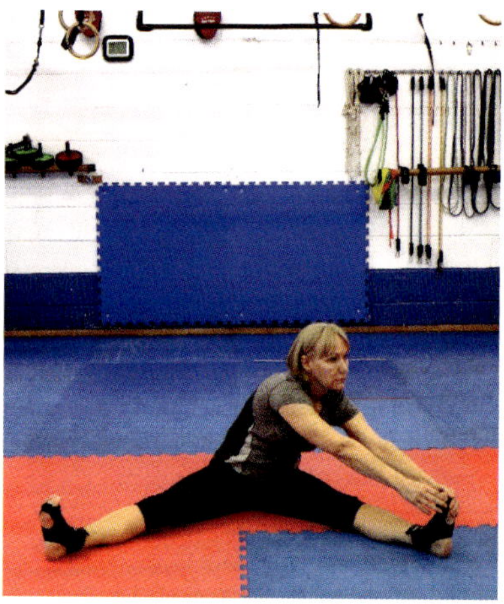

Figure 140

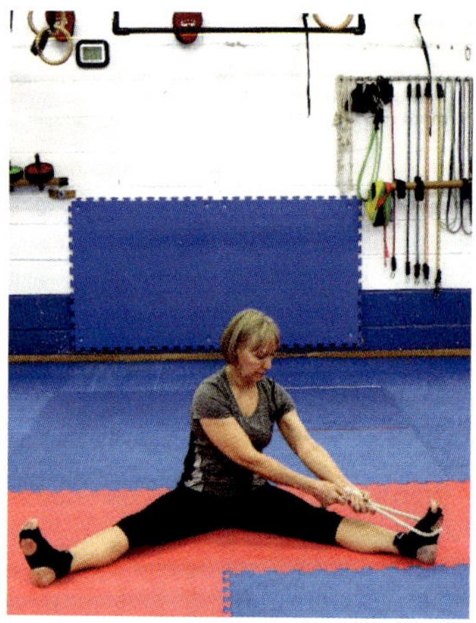

Figure 141

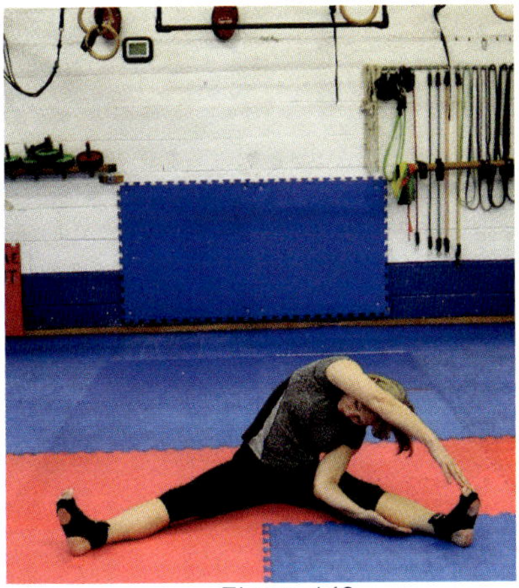

Figure 142

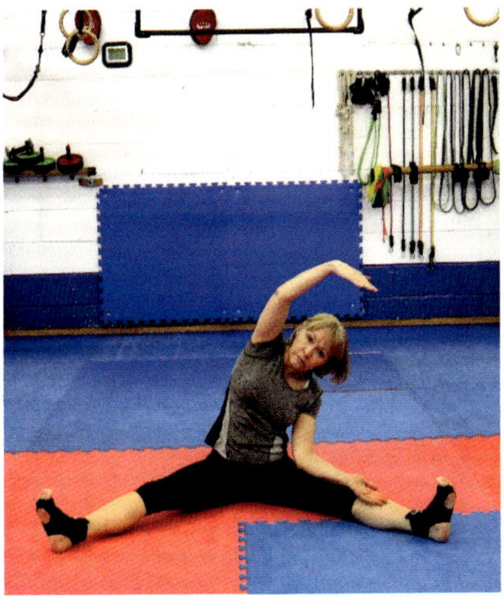

Figure 143

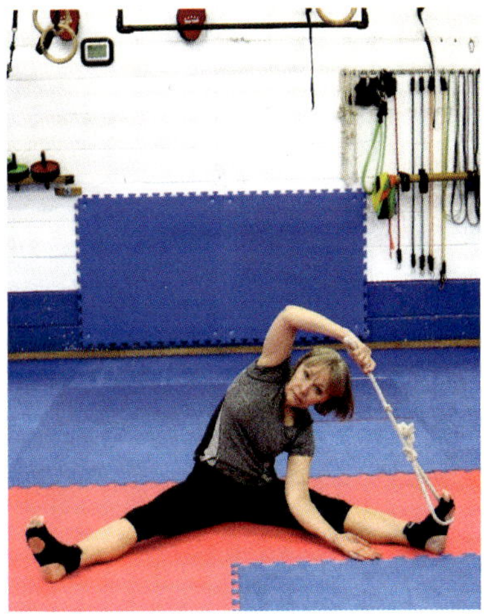

Figure 144

- Repeat the full sequence by lowering your body over your right leg. Reach your right foot with both hands, keeping your chin up ***(Figure 145)***. If you can't reach your right foot with your hands, use a rope or towel ***(Figure 146)***. Breathe out and hold for 10-15 seconds.
- Keep hold of your foot with your left hand, move your right elbow to the inside of your right knee palm facing up, and gently twist your body to the right by pulling and bringing your head down towards your right knee ***(Figure 147)***. Breathe out and hold for 10-15 seconds. If you can't reach your right foot with your hands there are two alternate ways to do this stretch ***(Figures 148 & 149)***.

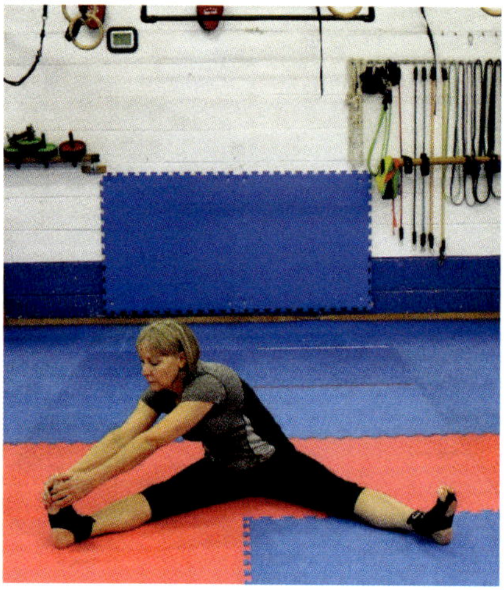

Figure 145

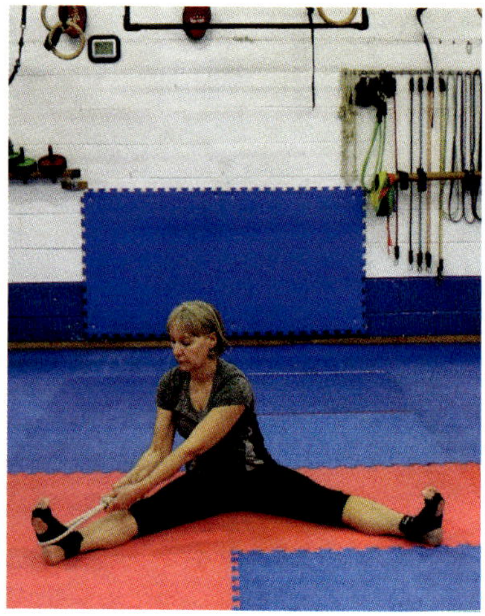

Figure 146

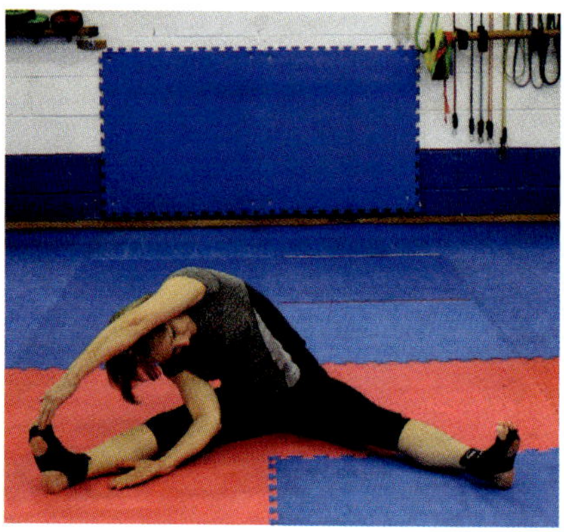

Figure 147

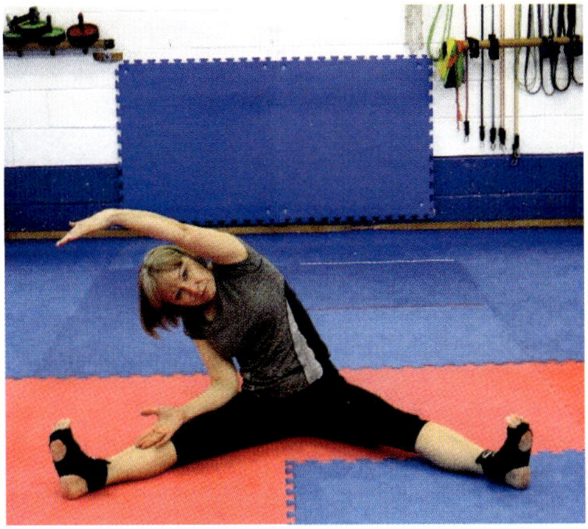

Figure 148

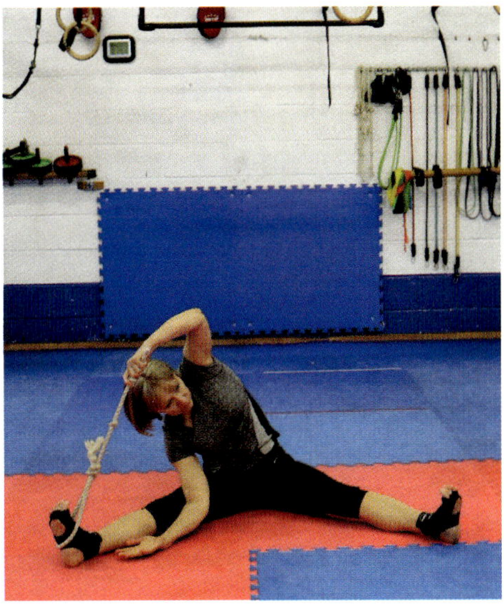

Figure 149

- Return to sitting position with legs together straight out in front of you and once more reach and stretch with both hands. Hold for 10-15 seconds ***(Figure 150).***
- Bend your left leg by pulling your left foot inside your right thigh, keeping your right leg straight in front of you ***(Figure 151)***. Reach with both hands over to your right foot. ***(Figure 152)***. Breathe out and hold for 10-15 seconds. If you cannot reach your foot, use a rope or towel ***(Figure 153)***.

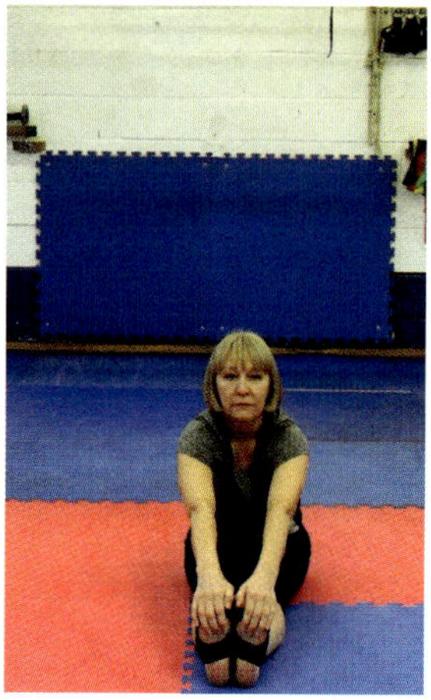

Figure 150

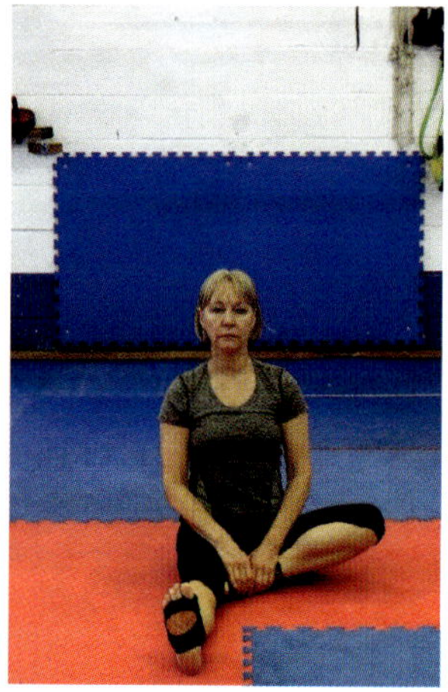

Figure 151

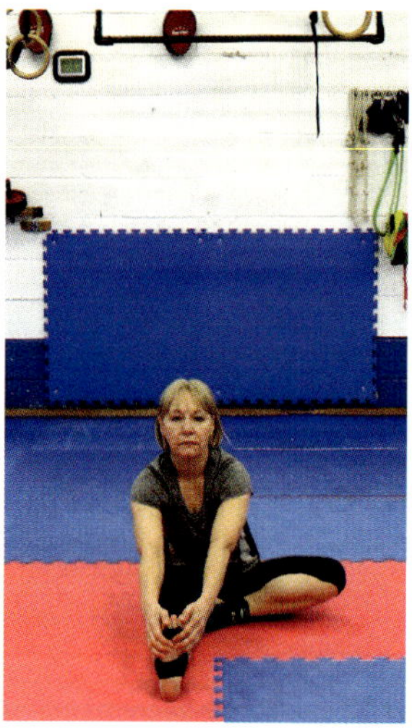

Figure 152

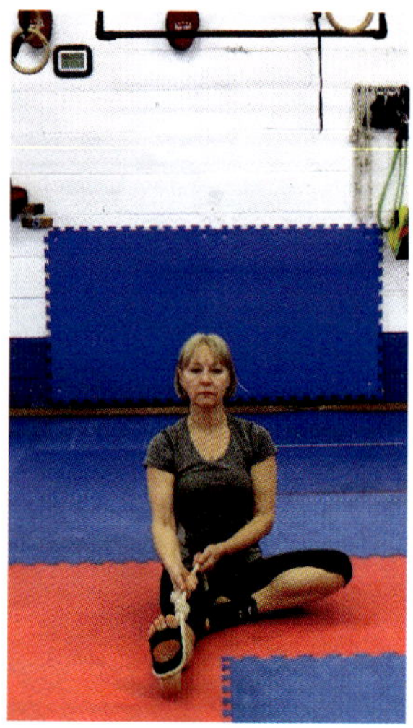

Figure 153

- Repeat the stretch over the left leg. Bend your right leg and pull your right foot inside your left thigh, keeping your left leg straight in front of you ***(Figure 154)***. Reach with both hands over to your left foot ***(Figure 155)***. Breathe out and hold for 10-15 seconds. If you can't reach your foot, use a rope or towel ***(Figure 156)***.

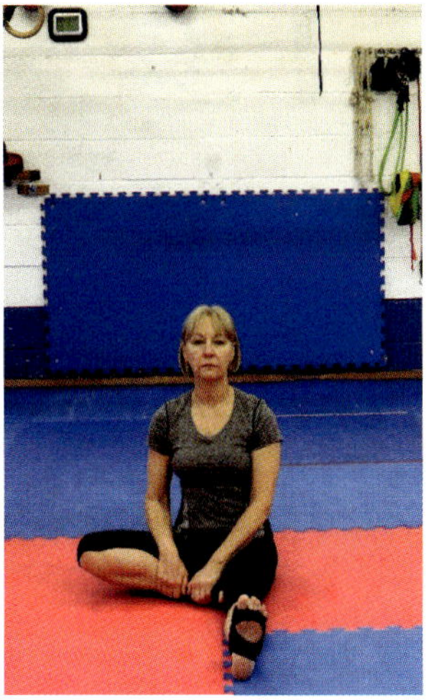

Figure 154

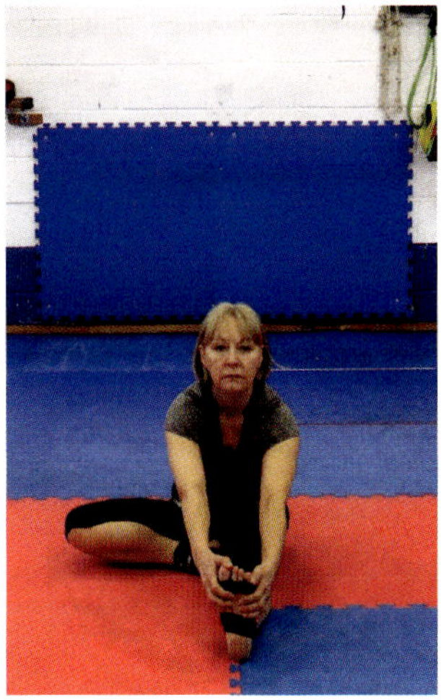

Figure 155

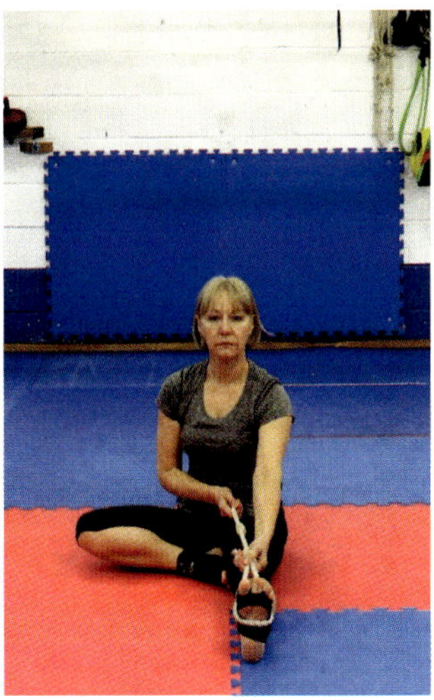

Figure 156

- Keep your right leg bent, bend your left leg and put both feet together. Grab hold of both feet with your hands, try to lower your knees to the floor and lower your body over your feet ***(Figure 157)***. Breathe out and relax for 10-15 seconds. If you cannot achieve this stretch use this alternate position ***(Figure 158)***.

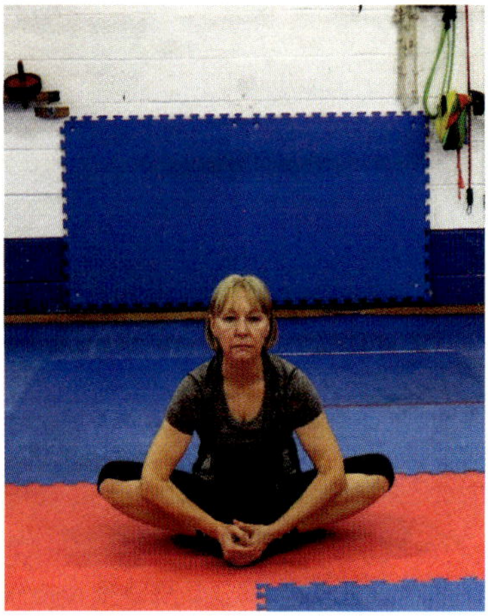

Figure 157

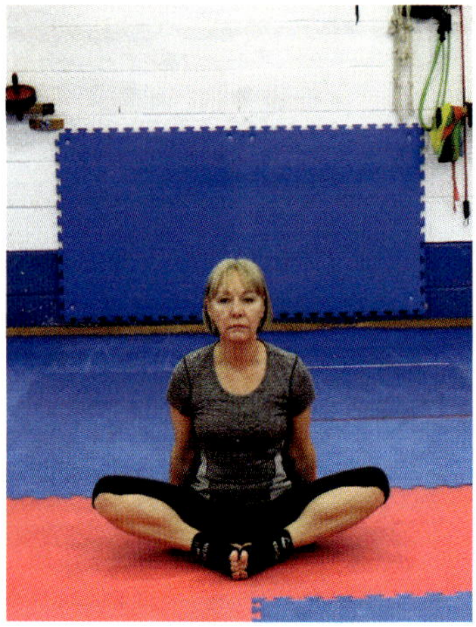

Figure 158

- Keeping your left leg bent in front of you and supporting yourself on your arms, move your right leg straight out behind you so that you are now half lying on the floor. Stretch your toes out and gently push your right hip to the floor. Straighten your arms up and arch your body. ***(Figures 159 / Figure160 side view)***. Hold for 10-15 seconds.

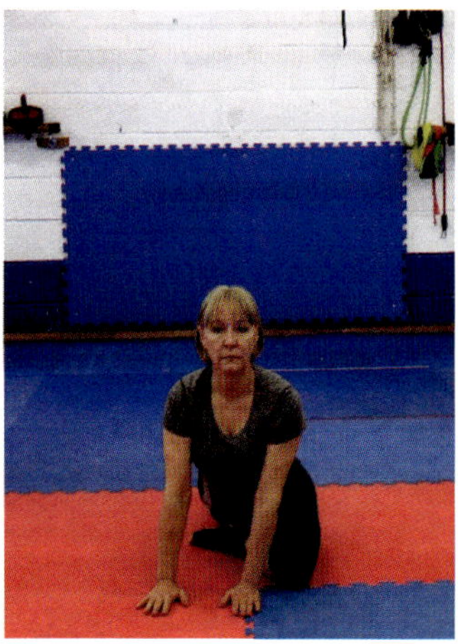

Figure 159

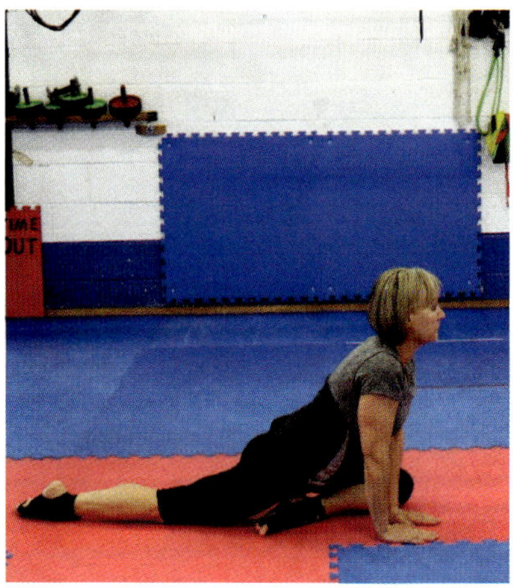

Figure 160 (side view)

- Repeat the same stretch to the other side with your right leg bent in front of you and left leg straight behind you ***(Figures 161 / Figure 162 side view)***. Breathe out and relax for 10-15 seconds.

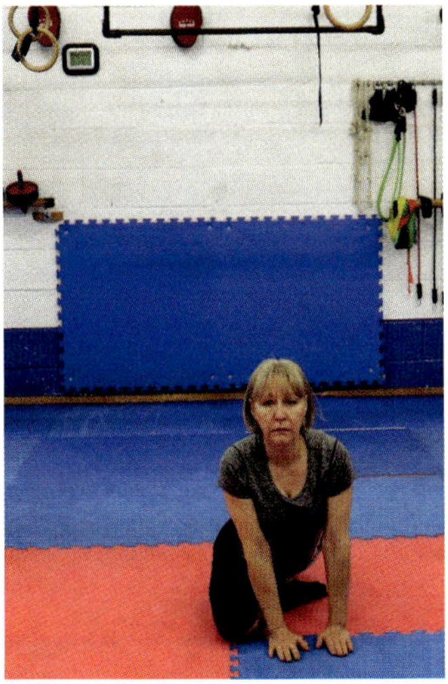

Figure 161

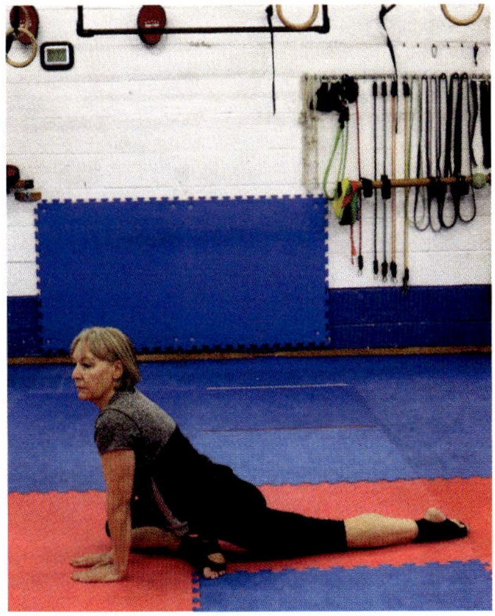

Figure 162 (side view)

- Straighten both legs out behind you and lay down on the floor, with your hands and forearms resting on the floor and your palms below your chest. Your big toes should be close together and every toenail should be on the floor ***(Figure 163 side view).*** Breathe out and relax for 10-15 seconds.
- Push your body up until you straighten your arms fully ***(yoga cobra position)*** and relax your hips by keeping them on the floor, knees also on the floor and toes stretched out behind you ***(Figure 164 side view).*** Breathe out and relax for 10-15 seconds. If your lower back is strong, the knees can be off the floor ***(Figure 165 side view)***.

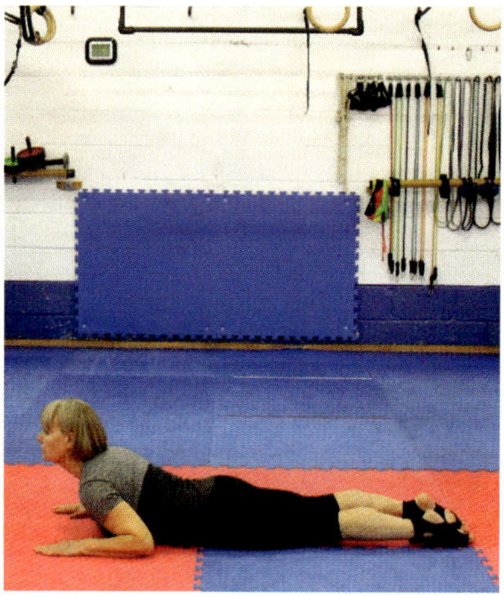

Figure 163 (side view)

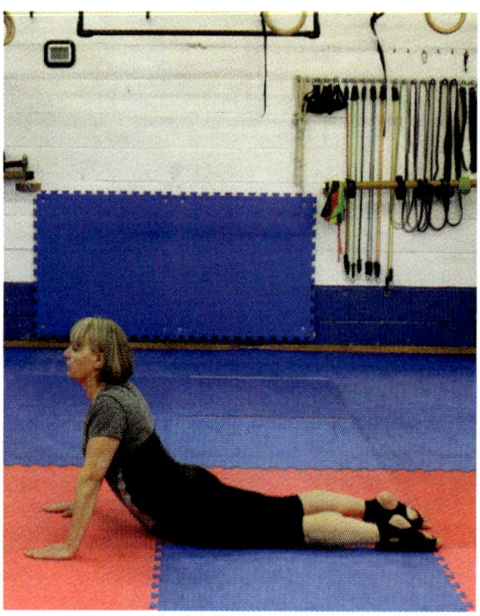

Figure 164 (side view)

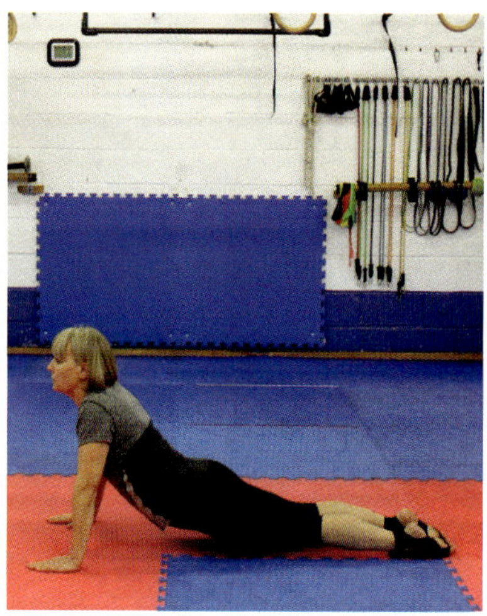

Figure 165 (side view)

- Now move your whole body back and sit over your legs, bottom resting on your feet and your hands straight out in front of you ***(yoga child pose position) (Figure 166 side view).*** Breathe out and relax for 10-15 seconds.

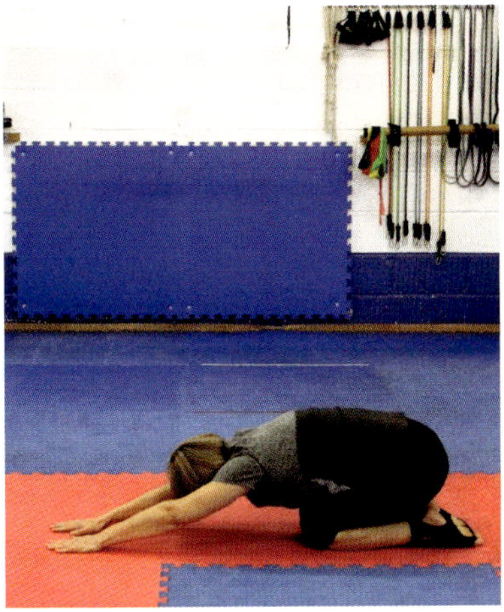

Figure 166 (side view)

- Open your feet a bit wider than your hips and gently lower your body backwards trying to lie down on your back ***(Figure 167 side view).*** If you are unable to perform this stretch you can either rest on your elbows or rest on your palms with arms straight ***(Figures 168 & 169 side view)***. Breathe out and relax for 10-15 seconds.

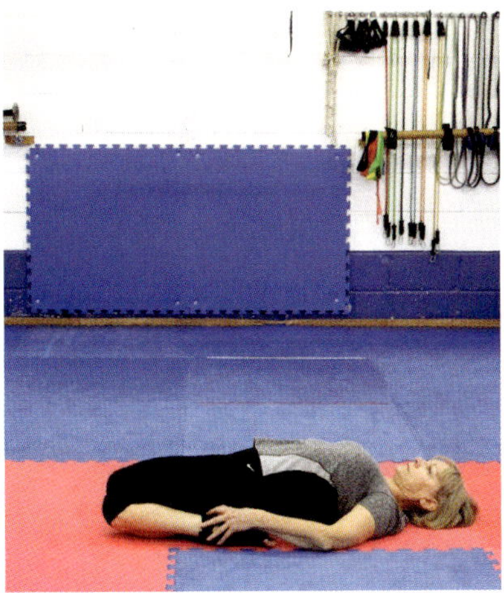

Figure 167 (side view)

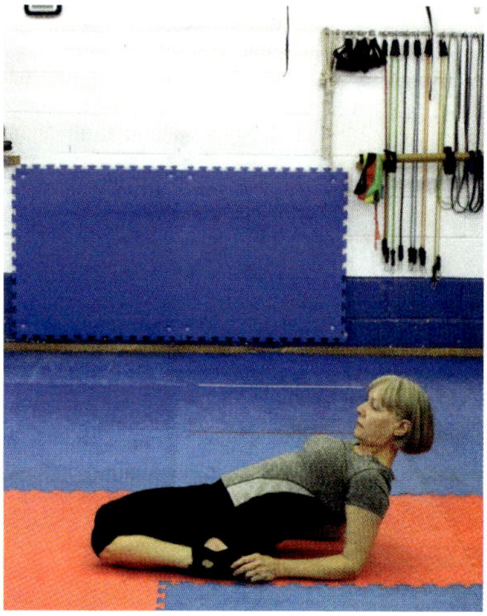

Figure 168 (side view)

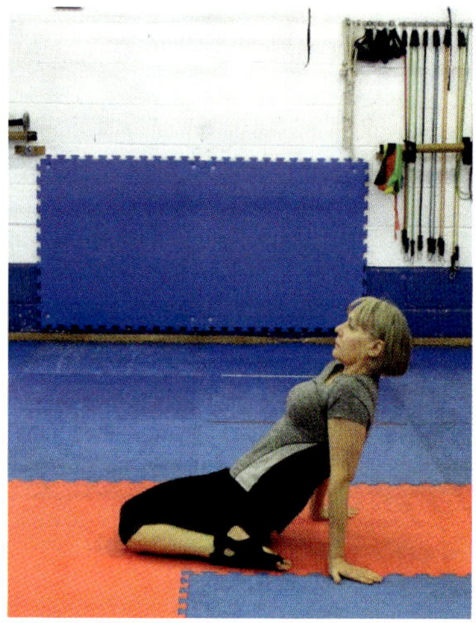

Figure 169 (side view)

- Raise your body up and remain in a kneeling position, your palms flat on the floor ***(yoga cat position) (Figure 170)***.
- Now open your knees wide apart, keeping both feet close together ***(Figure 171).***

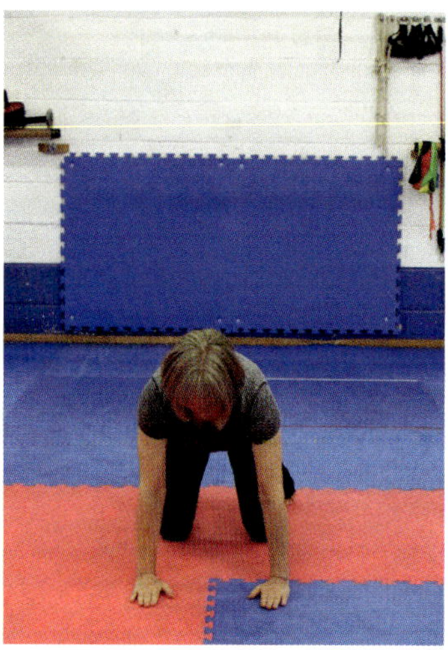

Figure 170

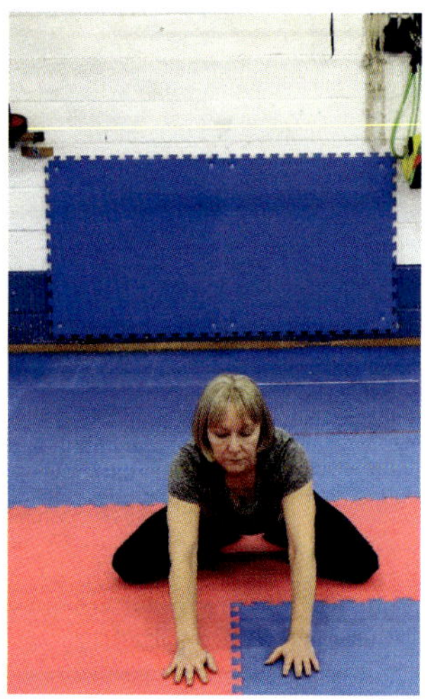

Figure 171

- Push your hips back until your bottom touches and rests over your feet, keeping your arms straight out in front of you. Relax your body to the floor in between your knees ***(Figure 172)***. Breathe out and relax for 10-15 seconds.
- Move your body forward, keeping your arms on the floor and widen your knees a bit more ***(Figure 173).***
- Move your body over your left leg. Breathe out and relax for 10-15 seconds ***(Figure 174)***.
- Repeat the stretch over your right leg. Breathe out and relax for 10-15 seconds ***(Figure 175).***

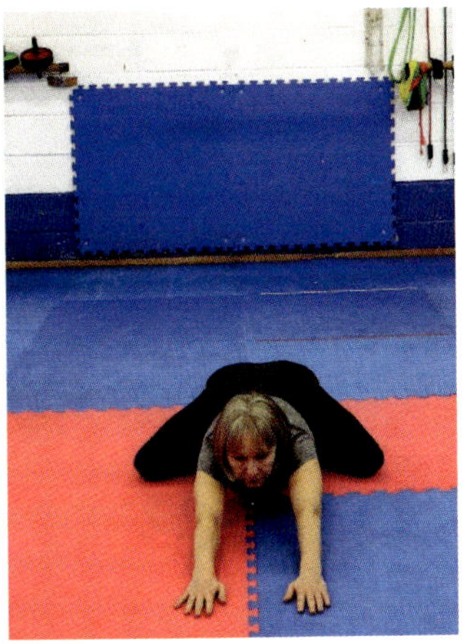

Figure 172

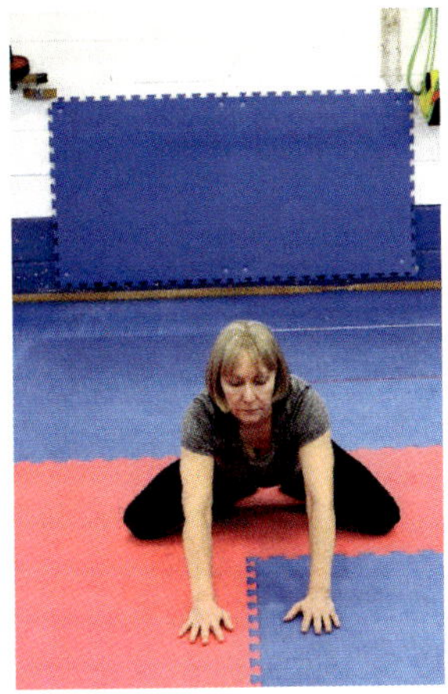

Figure 173

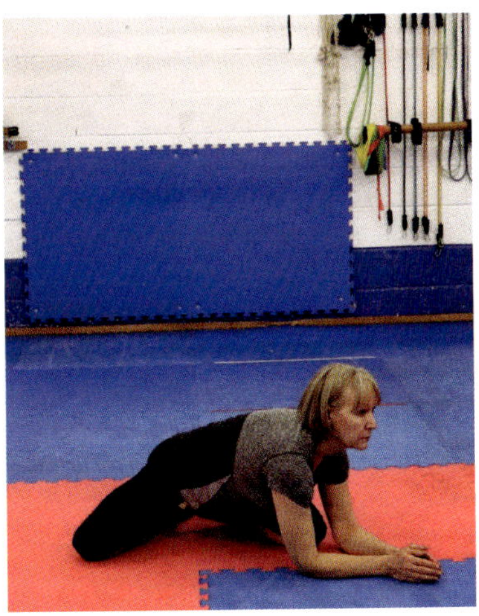

Figure 174

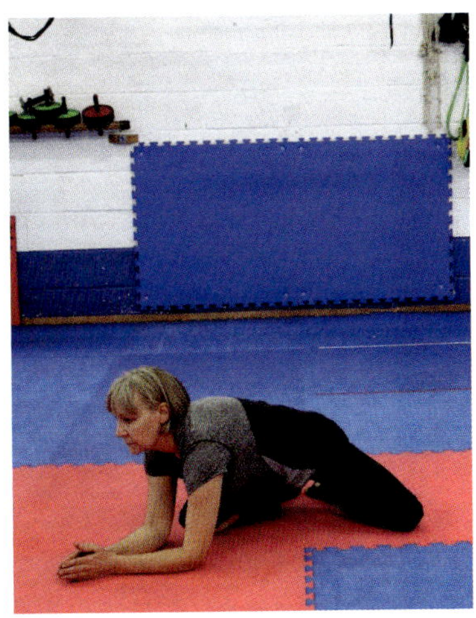

Figure 175

- Return your body to centre position, keeping your knees wide apart and both feet close together hands on the floor ***(Figure 176).***

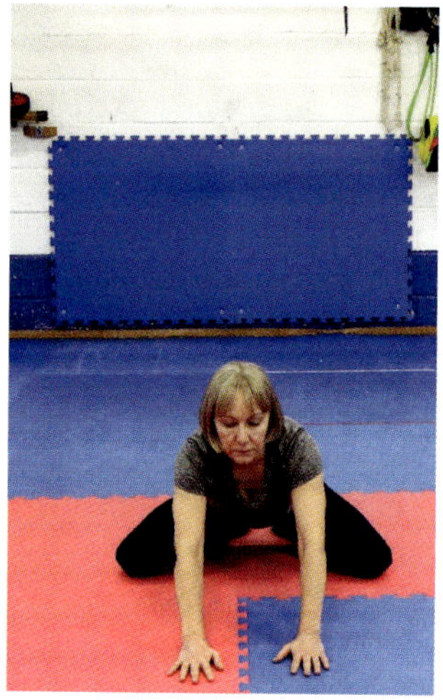

Figure 176

- Stretch your left hand in front of your chest and bend your right arm up above your left elbow. Stretch your left arm by twisting your body over to the right side ***(Figure 177)***. Breathe out and relax for 10-15 seconds.
- Repeat to the other side, with your right arm straight and your left arm bent above the right elbow ***(Figure 178).*** Breathe out and relax for 10-15 seconds.

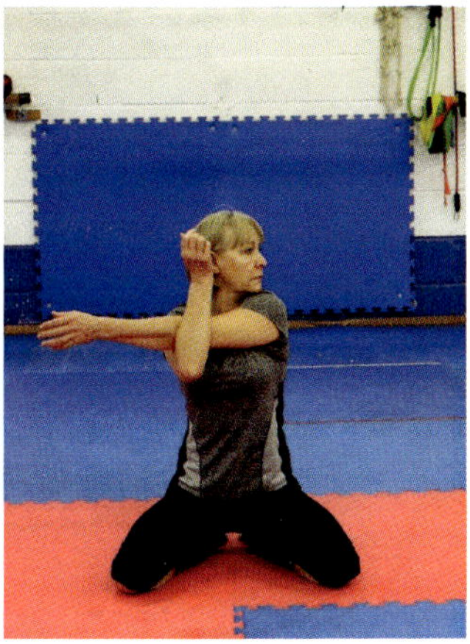

Figure 177

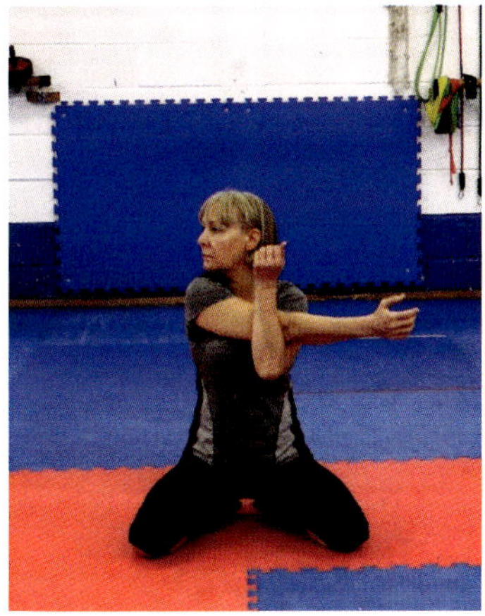

Figure 178

- Bend your left arm above your head and reach your right hand over to your left elbow. Gently push your left arm behind your head and lean your body over to your right-hand side ***(Figure 179).*** Breathe out and relax for 10-15 seconds.
- Repeat the same stretch to the other side with your right arm above and behind your head, your left arm holding the right elbow ***(Figure 180).*** Breathe out and relax for 10-15 seconds.

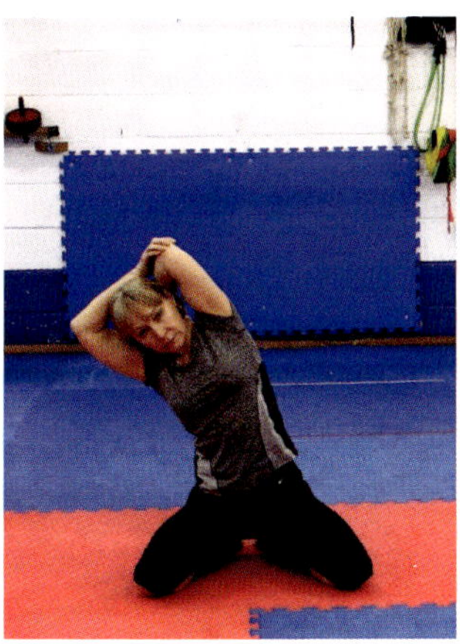

Figure 179

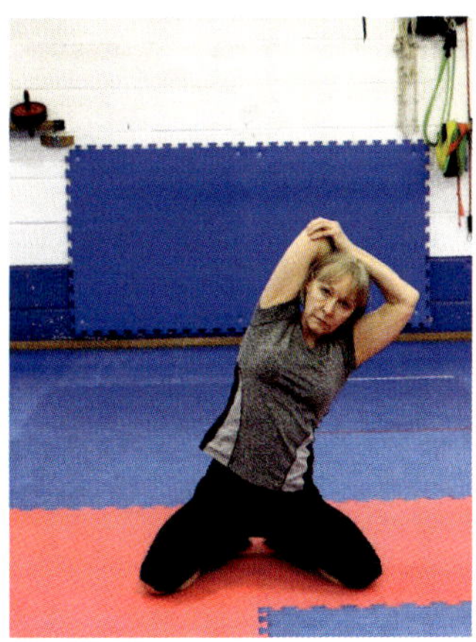

Figure 180

- Return to ***yoga cat position*** with your hands resting on the floor in front of you. Pull your knees together with your legs at 45 degrees from your body ***(Figure 181)***.

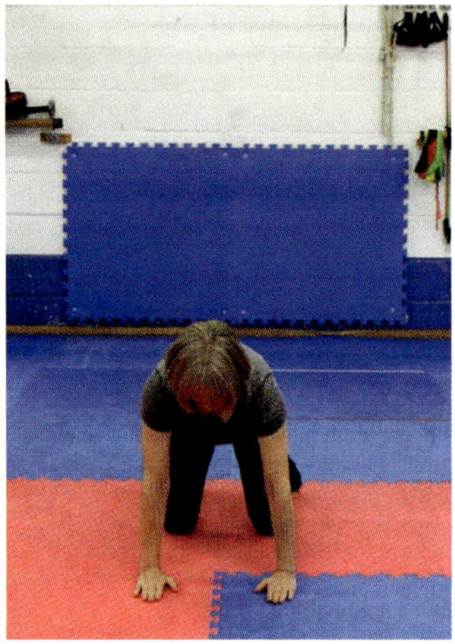

Figure 181

- Now elevate your knees until your legs are straight, keeping your heels off the floor, your arms straight and your head between your hands ***(Figure 182 side view)***.

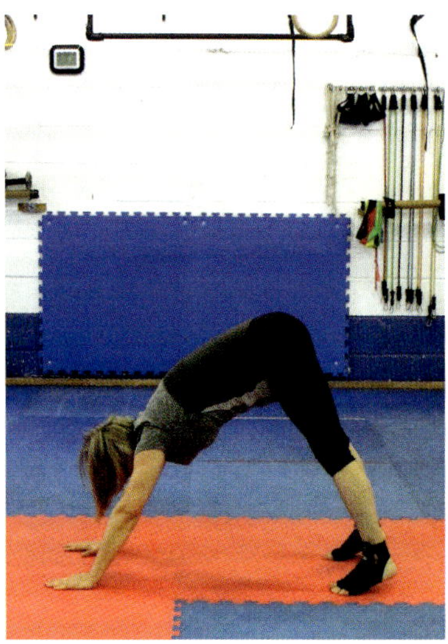

Figure 182 (side view)

- Gently push your chest towards your feet and stretch your shoulders towards your hips, lower your heels onto the floor ***(yoga downward dog position) (Figure 183 side view).*** Breathe out, relax and hold the stretch for 10-15 seconds.
- Move your palms to your toes ***(Figure 184 side view)***. Breathe out, relax and hold the stretch for 10-15 seconds.
- Now hug your legs round the back of your knees with both hands ***(Figure 185 side view)***. Breathe out, relax and hold the stretch for 10-15 seconds.

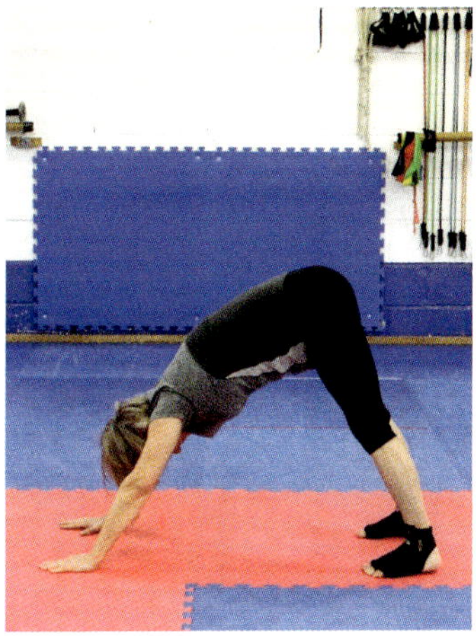

Figure 183 (side view)

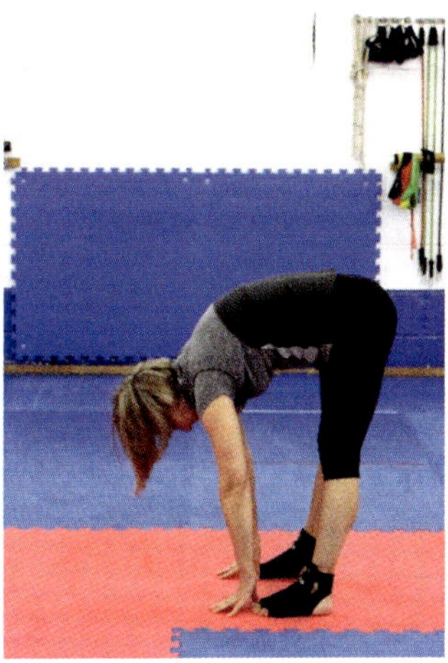

Figure 184 (side view)

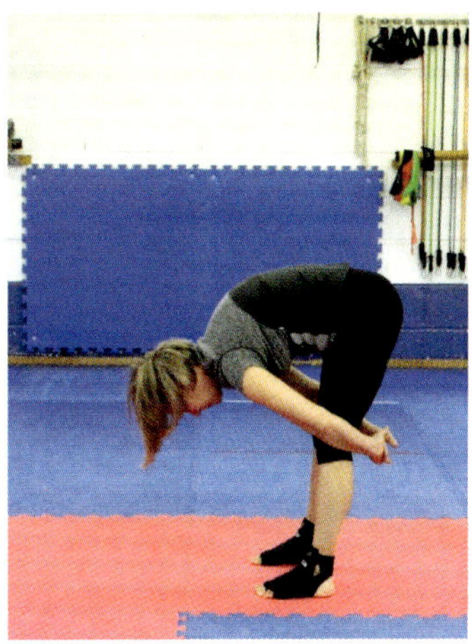

Figure 185 (side view)

- Free your hands, squat gently to half way up and put your hands on your knees ***(Figure 186 side view)***, then elevate your body up to a standing position ***(Figure 187).***
- Lift your arms out in front of you, shoulder height, with palms facing upwards. Swing your hands up over to your left shoulder, twisting at the waist and raising the heel off the ground when turning. Follow your arms with your eyes, raising both hands over the left shoulder (***Figure 188 side view***).
- Repeat over to the right shoulder ***(Figure 189 side view).***
- Lower your hands down to the hips and repeat the move, turning first over to the left hip ***(Figure 190)*** and then over the right hip ***(Figure 191).***
- Repeat this exercise 4 times.

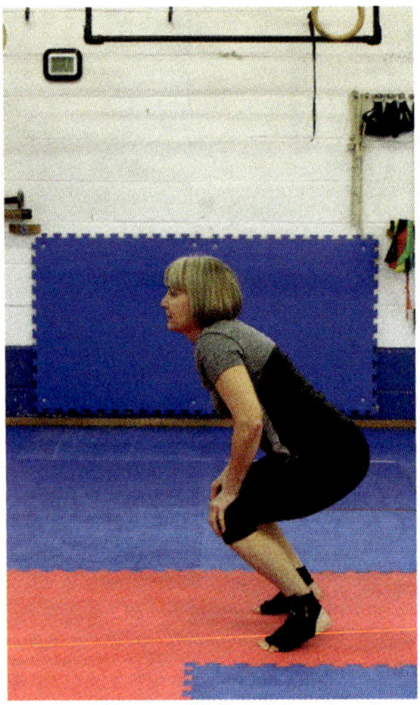

Figure 186 (side view)

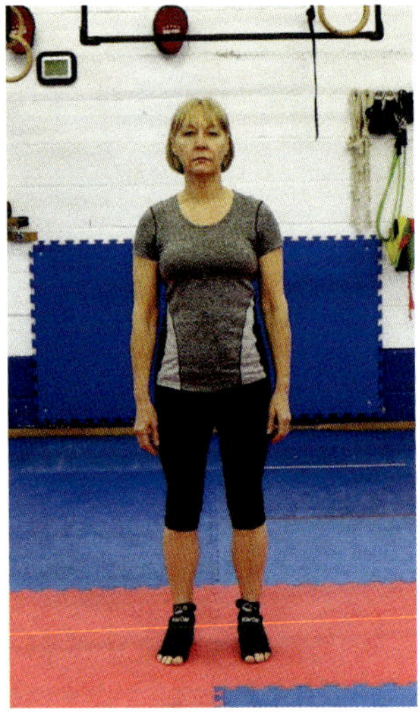

Figure 187

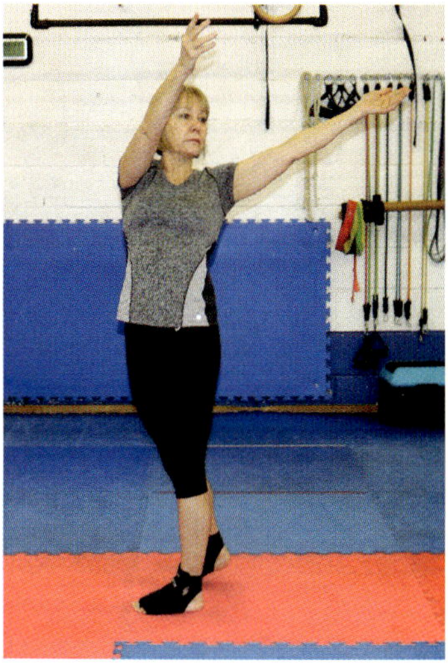

Figure 188 (side view)

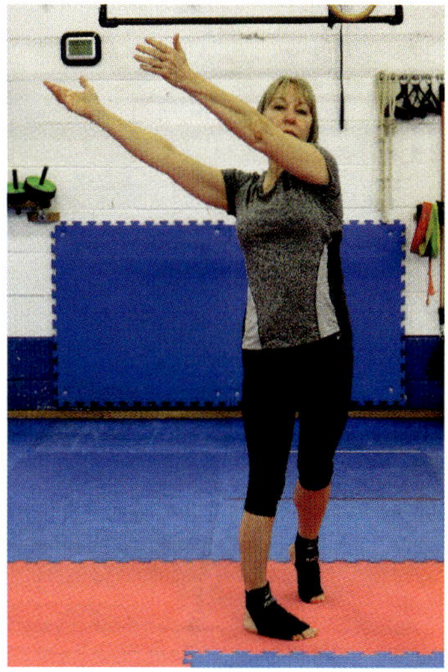

Figure 189 (side view)

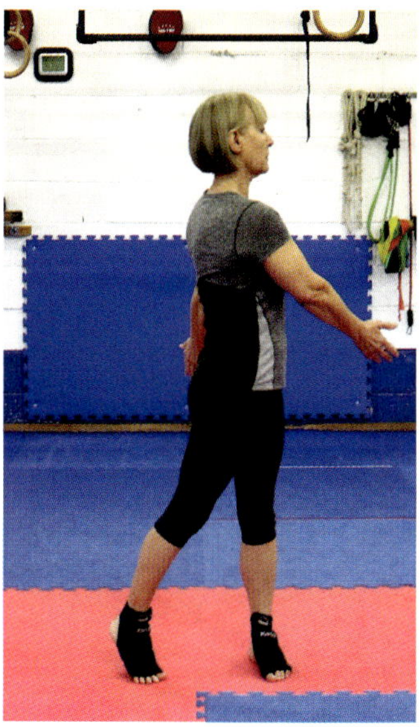

Figure 190

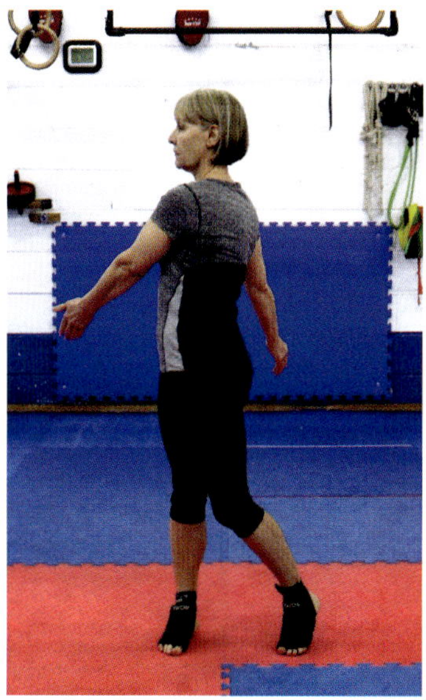

Figure 191

Well done. You have completed your first full programme and made your first big step towards putting your OA in REMISSION.

FOOD AND NUTRITION

(excerpt from *www.Verywellhealth.com*)

Anti-inflammatory diet

The anti-inflammatory diet is an eating plan designed to prevent or reduce low-grade chronic inflammation, a key risk factor in a host of health problems and several major diseases. The typical anti-inflammatory diet emphasises fruits, vegetables, lean protein, nuts, seeds and healthy fats.

Often resulting from lifestyle factors such as stress and lack of exercise, chronic inflammation results when the immune system releases chemicals meant to combat injury and bacterial and virus infections, even when there are no foreign invaders to fight off.

Since our food choices influence the level of inflammation in our bodies, an anti-inflammatory diet may be beneficial in curbing chronic inflammation and may also help prevent or treat the following conditions: allergies, Alzheimer's disease, arthritis, asthma, cancer, depression, diabetes, gout, heart diseases, inflammatory bowel diseases (such as ulcerative colitis and Crohn's disease), irritable bowel syndrome (IBS) and stroke.

Foods to eat on the anti-inflammatory diet

Research suggests that people with a high intake of vegetables, fruits, nuts, seeds, heathy oils and fish may have a reduced risk of inflammation-related diseases. In addition, substances found in some foods (especially antioxidants and omega-3 fatty acids) appear to possess anti-inflammatory effects. Food high in antioxidants include:

- Berries (such as blueberries, raspberries and blackberries)
- Cherries
- Apples
- Banana
- Artichokes
- Ginger root
- Avocados
- Dark green leafy vegetables (such as kale, spinach and collard greens)
- Sweet potatoes
- Broccoli
- Nuts (such as walnuts, almonds, pecans and hazelnuts)
- Beans (such as red beans, pinto beans and black beans)
- Whole grains (such as oats and brown rice)
- Dark chocolate (at least 70% cocoa)
- Foods high in omega-3 acids: oily fish (salmon, herring, mackerel, sardines and anchovies), flaxseeds, walnuts
- Omega-3-fortified foods: eggs and milk

It is believed that certain culinary herbs and spices such as ginger, turmeric and garlic may also help alleviate inflammation.

Foods to avoid

Omega-6 fatty acids (a type found in a range of foods) are known to increase the body's production of inflammatory chemicals. Since omega-6 acids help maintain bone health, regulate metabolism and promote brain function, you shouldn't cut them out of your diet altogether. However, it's important to balance your intake of omega-6 fatty acids with your intake of omega-3 fatty acids in order to keep inflammation in check.

Foods high in omega-6 fatty acids include:

- Meat
- Dairy products (such as milk, cheese, butter and ice cream)
- Margarine
- Vegetable oils (such as corn, soybean, peanut)
- Processed food

Instead of vegetable oils, opt for oils such as olive oil and avocado oil.

Additionally, studies show that a high intake of high-glycemic index foods such as white bread and many processed foods may increase inflammation. Avoid sugary drinks, refined carbohydrates, desserts, and processed snack foods.

My personal diet and food recipes

I am including some of my favourite recipes here in the hope that you will find them enjoyable too. Throughout the day I drink tap water but in the evening I regularly drink green tea with lemon and ginger, a recipe I also include here.

Breakfast

Serves 1

50g organic almonds
40g organic pumpkin seeds
20g organic sunflower seeds
10g organic sesame seeds
1 x banana
100g USN Anabolic protein powder
Still cold water

Put all ingredients except the protein powder into a 500ml (1pt) smoothie maker glass. Top it up with still tap water and lastly put the anabolic protein powder in. Mix together until all nuts, seeds and banana are well mashed.

Evening: Green Tea with Lemon & Ginger ice cube

Lemon & Ginger ice cubes
200g ginger root
4 fresh lemons

To prepare the ice cubes
Peel the ginger root and cut into fine slices. Cut the lemons in half and squeeze out the juice. Put the lemon juice and ginger root in a blender until puréed, adding more lemon juice or a little cold water if too dry.
Put into ice cube trays and freeze.

To make the tea
1 lemon & ginger ice cube
1 green tea bag
1 cup hot water

Put the tea bag in the hot water and add the ice cube. Stir during drinking.

Lunch / dinner recipes

Beetroot & feta or goat cheese salad with tuna
Serves 1

1 tin of tuna in spring water, drained
4 thin slices of feta or goats' cheese
1 small ball of pickled beetroot, sliced or chopped
Handful of rocket salad
1 tablespoon extra-virgin olive oil
1-2 tablespoons balsamic vinegar

Using a good-sized salad bowl, put the rocket salad in first.
Add the beetroot and the tuna chunks.
Sprinkle the oil and the vinegar over the bowl and lay the cheese on top.
Serve cold.

Five beans super food salad with Honey & Mustard dressing
Serves 1

1 tin (400g) of 5 bean salad in water (or you can use dried beans that you have soaked)
½ small red onion, chopped
100g of mixed leaves
5 cherry tomatoes
¼ cucumber, diced
10 olives

Dressing
30g Dijon mustard (or wholegrain if you prefer)
80g of honey
80g mayonnaise
1 tablespoon malt vinegar (or Apple Cider Vinegar)
¼ teaspoon cayenne pepper (or some dried chili flakes)
Put all the ingredients in a bowl and whisk until incorporated.

Assemble the salad by putting the mixed leaves in a bowl and adding the cucumber, tomatoes, onion, beans and olives.
Drizzle the dressing over the salad.

Serve cold.

Macedonian cabbage salad
Serves 1

¼ fresh cabbage
½ cucumber
1 tablespoon extra-virgin oil
1 tablespoon balsamic vinegar

Grate the cabbage using a small hole on the grater or chop finely.
Sprinkle the oil and vinegar over and mix well.
Cut the cucumber into thin slices and spread them around the outside of the salad.
Serve cold.

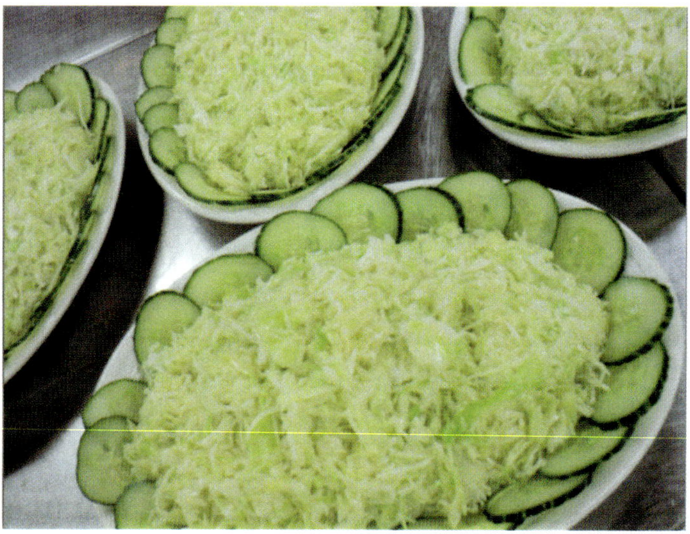

Salmon and broccoli
(Source: BBC Food)
Serves 1

150g wild salmon (fresh from a fish counter)
1 teaspoon virgin olive oil
2 lemon segments
½ teaspoon turmeric
½ teaspoon ground black pepper
100g (6-7 pieces) broccoli
1 teaspoon ground garlic

Pre-heat oven to 200C/180C Fan/Gas mark 5.
Put the salmon on aluminum foil. Spread the olive oil over the salmon followed by the turmeric and black pepper.
Place the lemon on the top of the salmon and wrap the aluminum foil closely over the salmon so that the cooking juices stay in the foil.
Place on a baking tray and bake for approximately 25-30min till cooked.
Towards the end of the cooking time, put the broccoli in a saucepan of boiling water with the ground garlic added. Cover and cook for 3-5 minutes, depending on how crunchy you like your broccoli.
Remove the salmon from the aluminum foil and place on warmed serving plates with the drained broccoli.
Serve hot.

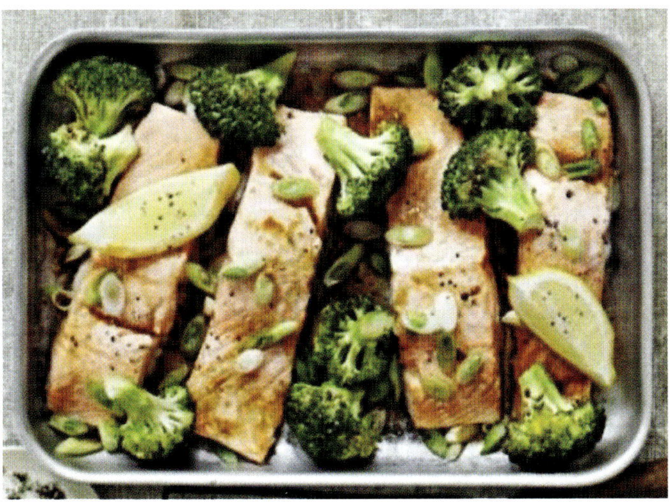

Mammas Lentils (serve as a meal, not a side dish)
Serves 2

100g brown or green lentils
1 onion, finely chopped
1 x carrot, finely chopped
1 teaspoon turmeric
½ teaspoon ground black pepper
½ teaspoon sea salt
1 tablespoon red paprika powder
1 x chicken breast (optional)
1 teaspoon hot chili powder (optional)
50mls cooking oil

Put the chicken breast in a medium-sized pan, cover with water, put the lid on and simmer on the hob until it is cooked.
Drain the chicken and then add the lentils to the pan. Fill with water to approx. ¾ full.
Add the onions and the remaining ingredients and stir well.
Cover with a saucepan lid and cook on the hob on a medium heat for approximately 45 minutes, stirring every 5 minutes to ensure it does not boil dry or stick to the pan.
If the water has reduced too much, add a little more as necessary.
Test the lentils after 30 minutes to check consistency.
The dish is ready to serve when the lentils are soft enough to eat.
Serve hot.

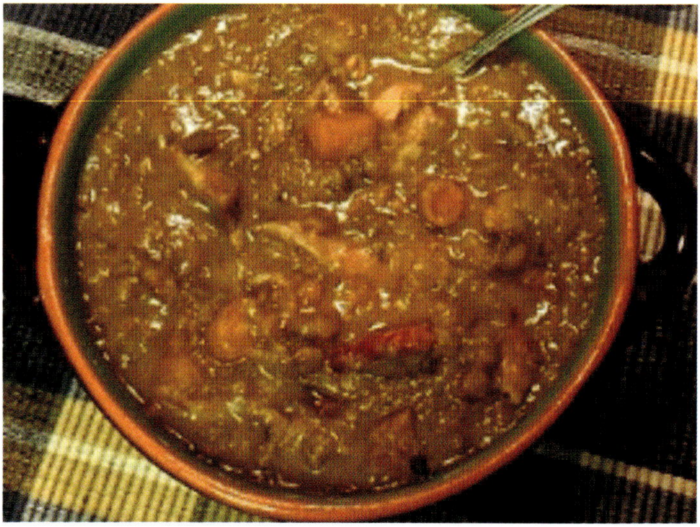

Baked Kale & Sardines
Serves 2

300g organic curly kale
handful of large green olives
2 tins of sardines or mackerel, drained
extra-virgin olive oil
garlic granules

Pre-heat oven to 200C/180C Fan oven/ Gas mark 5.

Put the kale on a baking sheet, sprinkle with the olive oil and garlic granules and put in the oven for 5 minutes.
Remove from oven and put on warmed serving plates.
Add the olives and sardines/mackerel to the kale.
Serve hot.

Macedonian beans in a pan
Serves 4

200g dried haricot beans (you can use butter beans, pinto beans or cannellini beans or a mix of these)
1 onion
1 clove fresh organic garlic
50mls cooking oil (sunflower oil)
1 teaspoon turmeric
½ teaspoon black pepper
½ teaspoon sea salt
1 tablespoon red paprika powder
1 teaspoon hot chili powder (optional)

For best results, soak the beans in cold water overnight or for 10-12 hours before cooking.

Put all the ingredients in a deep, saucepan and fill to approx. ¾ with cold water. Stir well, cover pan with lid and cook on a hob on medium-low heat.
Check and stir well every 5 minutes to ensure there is enough liquid in the pan to cover the beans. If needed, add more boiling water.
Simmer for 35-40 minutes, or until beans are soft and cooked.
When they are soft, remove the lid and continue cooking until the liquid reduces.
Then transfer the beans into an ovenproof dish, put in a pre-heated oven and bake at 200C/180C Fan/Gas mark 5 to cook for approx. 15-20 minutes or until they are at the consistency you prefer. (I like mine quite runny but my wife likes them drier!)
Serve hot.

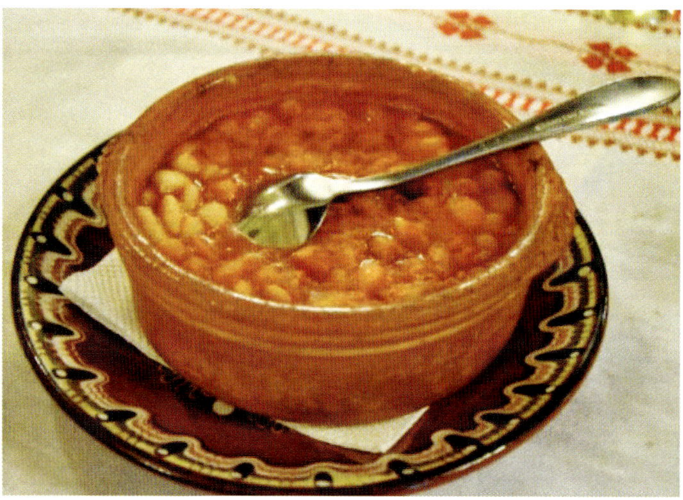

Spinach and kale on rice

Serves 4

100g brown rice
3 medium-sized onions, finely chopped
½ kg organic spinach
½ kg curly kale
100mls cooking oil (sunflower oil)
1 teaspoon turmeric
1 teaspoon garlic granules/powder (or few cloves crushed fresh garlic)
1 teaspoon hot chili powder (optional)
½ teaspoon ground black pepper
1 teaspoon sea salt (optional)
1 tablespoon red paprika powder
4 free range or organic eggs

<u>Side dish</u>
250g natural Greek yogurt
½ avocado, medium size
2 sticks celery, finely chopped
Blend ingredients together in a blender.

Put the onions and rice in a deep frying pan or wok, add 100mls cooking oil (sunflower oil), turmeric, garlic, chili powder, black pepper, sea salt and red paprika powder.
Cook on a high heat until the onion starts caramelizing (5-10 mins approximately).
Add the kale and 300mls hot water, and continue cooking until the kale goes soft, then add the spinach and cook until the spinach softens. Add water if necessary so it doesn't dry before you finish cooking.
Take out of the frying pan/wok and put in an ovenproof dish. Cook at 200C/180C Fan/Gas mark 5 for 30-35 minutes. Check after 15-20 minutes and, if the water has reduced, add a little more and stir.
When the rice is fully cooked, break and add the eggs to the rice without breaking the yolks. Spoon a little cooking liquid over the eggs and put the pan back in the oven for another 10 minutes or until the eggs are cooked to your liking.

Serve hot with the side dish.

Roasted, Cheesy Broccoli
(Source: Errenskitchen)

Serves 4

350g broccoli
4 garlic cloves, peeled and thinly sliced
Extra virgin olive oil
½ teaspoon salt
½ teaspoon freshly ground black pepper
50g freshly grated Parmesan cheese (or your preferred cheese – I sometimes use Cheddar)

Preheat the oven to 200C/180C Fan/Gas mark 5.

Cut the broccoli florets from the thick stalks, leaving 2-3cm of stalk attached to the florets, discarding the rest of the stalks. Cut the larger pieces through the base of the head with a small knife, pulling the florets apart.
Place the florets on a baking sheet large enough to hold them in a single layer. Toss the garlic on the broccoli and drizzle with 5 tablespoons olive oil. Sprinkle with the salt and pepper.
Roast for 10 minutes until crisp but tender and the tips of some of the florets are browned.
Remove from the oven and add the parmesan (or other cheese) and put back in the oven for another 3 minutes.
Serve hot

This is lovely as a light lunch or I often add roasted chicken, grilled fish or a poached egg for my main meal!

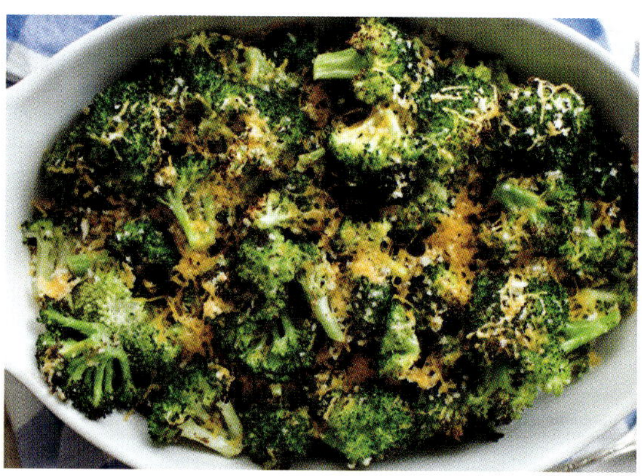

Tarragon-rubbed salmon with nectarine salsa

(Source: adapted from *Good Housekeeping*)

Serves 4

2 tablespoon red onion, finely chopped
2 large ripe nectarines, chopped
1 small red pepper, chopped
1 jalapeño chili pepper, finely chopped
2 tablespoon fresh lime juice
1 tablespoon chopped fresh parsley
½ teaspoon salt
¼ teaspoon coarsely ground black pepper
1 tablespoon dried tarragon
4 pieces skinless salmon fillet
1 teaspoon olive oil

<u>To make the salsa</u>
In medium bowl, mix finely chopped red onion, chopped nectarines, chopped red pepper, finely chopped jalapeño, lime juice, chopped parsley and ¼ teaspoon salt. Set aside.

<u>For the salmon</u>
In small bowl, combine tarragon, ¼ teaspoon salt, and ¼ teaspoon coarsely ground black pepper.
Brush salmon with oil and rub with tarragon mixture to coat both sides.
Place salmon in a hot frying pan. Cover pan and cook salmon 8 to 10 minutes or until it turns opaque throughout, turning over once with large spatula. Transfer to platter and serve with the salsa.
Serve hot.

I love steamed asparagus, and this is especially good with this dish or you could add boiled new potatoes for your main meal.

Peppercorn-crusted tuna with ginger and soy dressing
(Source: BBC Food)

Serves 2

115g jar green peppercorns in brine, drained and roughly chopped (you could use peppercorns in a grinder that most supermarkets sell as an easier/quicker alternative)
2 x 100g fresh tuna steaks
50mls olive oil
200g baby leaf spinach

<u>For the dressing</u>
1 tablespoon finely chopped ginger
½ bunch chives, finely chopped
100ml vegetable oil
1–2 tablespoon soy sauce
1 teaspoon sesame oil
1 garlic clove, crushed
1 lemon, juice only
salt and freshly ground black pepper
Put all the dressing ingredients into a screw-top jar and shake to combine, or, alternatively, whisk together in a small bowl. Season with salt and pepper.

Put the peppercorns in a shallow bowl and press the tuna steaks down onto them. Turn the steaks over and repeat on the other side.
Heat the olive oil in a large frying pan set over a high heat. Sear the tuna for 1–2 minutes on each side. Remove the tuna from the pan and set aside to rest. Add the spinach to the pan and cook, stirring, until wilted.

<u>To serve</u>
Divide the spinach between two serving plates. Slice the tuna steaks into three, lay on top of the spinach and dress with the ginger and soy dressing.

This is great for a light lunch or you can add rice or noodles for a filling and tasty dinner.

Red Lentil and Spinach Masala
(Source: feed me phoebe)

Serves 4

1 tablespoon olive or coconut oil
1 small red onion, diced
2 garlic cloves, minced
inch fresh ginger, peeled and minced
1 serrano chili pepper, seeded and minced
1 teaspoon ground cumin
1 teaspoon garam masala
¼ teaspoon coriander
1 x 425g can diced tomatoes
1 teaspoon sea salt
1 x 425mls can unsweetened full fat coconut milk
130g red lentils
150g baby spinach

In a large stock pot or Dutch oven, heat the oil. Sauté the onion over a medium-high heat until soft, approximately 5 minutes.
Add the garlic, ginger, serrano, cumin, garam masala, and coriander. Cook until very fragrant, approximately 2 minutes.
Carefully pour in the tomatoes and add the salt, scraping up any brown bits that formed on the bottom of the pan. Cook, stirring occasionally, until the liquid has reduced and the tomato chunks have softened, approximately 5 minutes.
Add the coconut milk and 250mls water. Bring to a boil over high heat.
Stir in the lentils and reduce the heat to medium-low. Cook until the lentils are tender, approximately 25-35 minutes, stirring occasionally to prevent the lentils from sticking to the bottom of the pan.
Fold in the spinach and cook until wilted, approximately 3 minutes.
For extra protein you could add chickpeas or chicken.

Serve with coconut rice or your favourite naan bread (mine is Peshwari) and some mango chutney.

About the Author

Kire Antoski was born in 1963 in Prilep, Northern Macedonia and grew up in a working-class family of four with his parents and younger sister. Having suffered bullying from local boys, he took up martial arts at the age of 13 when he joined a local Karate club. During his college years he was active in other sports, playing handball for the college team as well as playing basketball for the local club. After finishing college, Kire was recruited into the former Yugoslavian armed forces, undertaking 15 months' National Service in Croatia. In 1983, having completed his National Service, he returned to Prilep and rejoined his karate club, as well as joining the ju jutsu club. In 1985 Kire added kickboxing to his training. He was selected to join his karate club's semi-professional competition team, with whom he competed until he emigrated to Great Britain with his young family in June 1990.

Needing to provide for his family, he worked long hours in several different jobs whilst also studying English at Hammersmith College. In spring 1991, the screen-printing business in which he was employed was moved to Sherborne, Dorset and Kire was offered a managerial position if he was prepared to move his family to the south-west of England, an opportunity he was happy to take. He continued working as a screen printer and also took up a position as nightclub security in a Yeovil club.

Kire never lost his love for martial arts and trained by himself until January 1994, when he decided to open his own martial arts club, "Panthers", in the aerobic studio of the local gym, running a few evening classes weekly. In 1998 he founded his full-time martial arts school, "Panthers Martial Arts Academy" which is based in Yeovil, Somerset. He works there still as a full-time martial arts and fitness instructor. Kire has grown Panthers Martial Arts Academy to be one of the largest and most successful martial arts schools in Somerset with over 190 students, of which 15 hold World titles, 9 hold European titles and 40 hold British titles. In 2018 Kire was nominated for the Somerset "Coach of the Year" award.